CASE STUDIES IN
SPORT DIPLOMACY

CASE STUDIES IN SPORT DIPLOMACY

CRAIG ESHERICK
George Mason University

ROBERT E. BAKER
George Mason University

STEVEN JACKSON
University of Otago, New Zealand

MICHAEL SAM
University of Otago, New Zealand

EDITORS

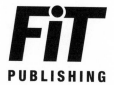

PUBLISHING

FiT Publishing
A Division of the International Center for Performance Excellence
West Virginia University
375 Birch Street, WVU-CPASS · PO Box 6116
Morgantown, WV 26506-6116
800.477.4348 (toll free) · 304.293.6888 (phone) · 304.293.6658 (fax)
Email: fitcustomerservice@mail.wvu.edu
Website: www.fitpublishing.com

Library of Congress Card Catalog Number: 2016957279

ISBN: 9781940067056

Cover Design: 40 West Studios
Cover Photos: © Libux77 | Dreamstime.com
Copyeditor: Geoff Fuller
Typesetter: Scott Lohr
Proofreader/Indexer: Eileen Harvey / Geoff Fuller
Printed by: Data Reproductions, Inc.

10 9 8 7 6 5 4 3 2 1

FiT Publishing
A Division of the International Center for Performance Excellence
West Virginia University
375 Birch Street, WVU-CPASS
PO Box 6116
Morgantown, WV 26506-6116
800.477.4348 (toll free)
304.293.6888 (phone)
304.293.6658 (fax)
Email: fitcustomerservice@mail.wvu.edu
Website: www.fitpublishing.com

TABLE OF CONTENTS

FOREWORD

In an era of such divisiveness, it behooves all of us to consider means by which we can bring people together. The concept of diplomacy through sports is one means, in particular, that I have championed. While serving as Deputy Secretary of State, I saw first-hand the power of sports diplomacy through the Department's use of CultureConnect Ambassadors, which brought recently graduated Georgetown University basketball players before young people throughout the world.

CultureConnect operated at a time of great unpopularity for the U.S. government. Our nation had recently invaded Afghanistan and Iraq, and the abuses perpetrated by U.S. service men and women at Abu Ghraib were coming to light. In the face of this negativity, these outstanding former basketball players, with their winning personalities, brought forward a new image of the U.S. They did not have to address the vexing foreign policy issues of the time. They were able to tell the story of America from their personal perspectives; a story that young children from across the world were interested in hearing. There was talk of basketball, but also of race relations, college life in the U.S., and cultural values. Our nation was so well-served by their efforts.

The story of CultureConnect is told in this well-researched book along with a number of other important case studies that bear witness to the value of sport diplomacy, as well as its limitations. The book's chapters delve into the range of sports related events that run the gamut from the "smart power" of individual participants to "mega projects," such as the Olympic Games. Together, the authors give us a sophisticated view of when and how sports diplomacy can be effective.

While we would all like to think of sport diplomacy as an absolute good, like any form of diplomacy, there is a nuance to it. The Olympic Games, for example, can be a double-edged sword for any host nation. On the one hand, they can signal a country's arrival on the world stage, such as with the Sochi Winter Games of 2014 or the Beijing Summer Games of 2008. On the other hand, they also can bring unwelcomed high-level international scrutiny to a nation's policies on such issues as homophobia, LGBT inequality, the environment, and human rights.

There is also a caution against sport diplomacy as a response to disaster. Haiti and South Sudan, after their many travails, had other priority needs before receiving stadiums – notwithstanding the many great Haitian and Sudanese athletes. And, perhaps the biggest caution of all surrounds the 1969 El Salvador-Honduras "soccer war;" when FIFA World Cup qualifying matches sparked actual conflict. Clearly, no amount of sport diplomacy can reverse underlying territorial issues or class tensions as was seen then in Central America and is now observed on the Korean Peninsula.

Messrs. Esherick, Baker, Jackson, and Sam have done us all a great service in bringing these important ideas forward. Sport diplomacy is a tremendous part of our nation's tool kit. How and when it is played, however, matters greatly. This book should be required reading for sport departments, government agencies involved in diplomacy, and for all those sports enthusiasts, like myself, who value international engagement.

– Mr. Richard Armitage
Former Deputy Secretary of State for the United States of America

PREFACE

This book is the result of many conversations the editors have had over the years with publishers, sport diplomats, and writers, all of whom recognized the need for a book like this to address the growing interest in the subject of sport diplomacy and the intersecting worlds of sports, politics, higher education, government, and diplomacy.

We recognize the power and ability of sport to accomplish different objectives on behalf of local communities, international sports organizations, for-profit sporting goods companies, and professional sports teams. Many books, papers and journal articles have chronicled the role of sport by non-profit, non-governmental organizations for a myriad of development objectives, most notably as a means of bringing peace to regions of the world that have faced conflict. The use of sport on behalf of governments for diplomatic purposes has not been as well documented. This book is an attempt to bring more of these efforts to light.

A talented and experienced group of writers have been asked to describe how sport is used for diplomatic purposes all over the world.

Bob Heere and Judit Trunkos set the stage, introducing the reader to the concept of sport diplomacy and its many iterations. In Chapter 2, Carrie LeCrom and Melissa Ferry discuss how the United States government and the US Department of State has used sports to further its influence around the world. In Chapter 3, Omari Faulkner, a sport diplomat himself, gives his insight into how the program, begun under the direction of U.S. Secretary of State Colin Powell, was managed. Paul Wright, Jenn Jacobs, Tim Ressler and Steven Howell discuss their efforts in the Belize Youth Sport Coalition, a part of the US Department of State Grants Program.

Scott Jedlicka, in Chapter 5, analyzes the International Olympic Committee (IOC) investment in a sports facility in the country of Haiti, debating whether this is diplomacy on behalf of the IOC or simply unadulterated capitalism.

In chapter six, seven, and eight our authors provide a fascinating look at the sports diplomacy efforts on behalf of three of the most influential governments in the world: Brazil, Russia, and China. Brazil's sport diplomacy is centered on mega-events (World Cup and Summer Olympics), China focuses their efforts on the building of sports facilities for trading partners, and Russia's sport diplomacy efforts are directed by Vladimir Putin.

In Chapter 9, Soolmaz Abooali breaks down the attempts by the United States and Iran to establish closer relations through the use of a sport that dates back to the very beginning of sport and the Olympic Games. In Chapter 10 Kyle Rich and Laura Misener discuss the impact of the Pride House movement in conjunction with the 2015 Pan Am Games in Toronto, Canada. In many ways this chapter parallels the discussion we see in Chapter 5: a diplomatic effort on behalf of an organization separate from a national government.

The final two chapters discuss sport diplomacy in countries on the continents of Asia and Africa. Myles Schrag outlines a strategy to leverage sports in South Sudan that would announce its independence, as well as foster a sense of national identity among its citizens. In Chapter 12, Ik Young Chang describes the many efforts the governments of North and South Korea have used to bring the two nations together through sport.

We hope the writers and their diverse discussions of sport diplomacy will motivate you to learn more and inspire you to get involved in sport diplomacy yourself.

– The Editors

ACKNOWLEDGMENTS

It has been a pleasure to work with such a talented group of writers to make this effort become a reality. I would like to acknowledge the hard work of my fellow editors and our colleagues at FiT Publishing. Finally, I want to thank the US Department of State and SportsUnited for the opportunity to work with some very talented athletes, coaches, and sports administrators from all over the world, engaging in our own version of sports diplomacy with my co-workers at George Mason University's Center for Sport Management.

–Craig Esherick

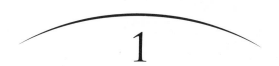

1

SPORT DIPLOMACY: A REVIEW OF HOW SPORTS CAN BE USED TO IMPROVE INTERNATIONAL RELATIONSHIPS

JUDIT TRUNKOS · BOB HEERE

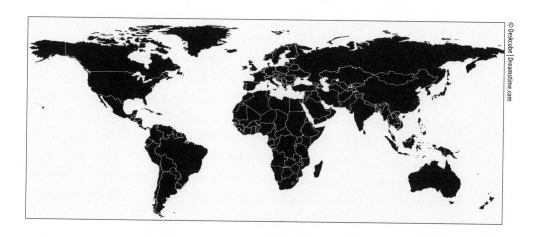

ABSTRACT

How can states leverage international sports events to strengthen their international relations? The emphasis in this discussion is on the instruments that states have at their disposal. *Sports diplomacy* falls under *public diplomacy,* which is used to improve intermediate and long-term relations between states by influencing the public abroad to accomplish foreign policy goals (Gilboa, 2008). Through a review of different foreign policy objectives that are common in multilateral diplomacy, we discuss the effectiveness of sports as a platform for diplomacy. The most common strategic objectives are (a) providing an unofficial reason and location for international leaders to meet and begin a dialogue; (b) providing insights into the host country and educating others about it; (c) bridging cultural and linguistic differences among nations and seeking common ground through sports; (d) creating a platform for new trade agreements or legislation; (e) creating awareness for the international relationship through sport ambassadors; (f) creating a legacy for the host country, improving its image in the world; and (g) using sport to provide legitimacy for a new nation.

UNDERSTANDING INTERNATIONAL RELATIONS

Countries interact on a daily basis and have ongoing dialogues on many issues, which include political, social, economic, and military problems. How they handle these issues and which foreign policy instruments they select to resolve potential problems or challenges is up to the leaders of the state. Realist scholarship has largely focused on military and economic capabilities, geography, natural resources, population, and political stability and competence in terms of sources of power. According to the Realist worldview, conflict is expected to happen between nations so the implementation of new and versatile diplomatic tools such as sport diplomacy is not their first choice of action. Realist scholars generally argue that power is mainly force and military strength (Morgenthau, 1948; Kissinger, 1994). Liberal scholars on the other hand, look into other aspects of power, including influence (Nye, 1990; Keohane & Nye, 2001). The Liberal approach is more interested in states' interaction during periods of peace than are the Realists. While force may be the obvious choice during conflict, during peacetime many new diplomatic tools can be considered. Liberal scholarship is thus concerned with alternative tools such as economic diplomacy, cyber diplomacy, and sports diplomacy. This book focuses on the application and evaluation of a specific diplomatic tool, namely *sports diplomacy*.

Diplomatic success stories, while they are very important, are usually not as noteworthy as military victories. One of the most well-known achievements of diplomacy is the Marshall Plan. This US-funded economic package jump-started the European economic recovery after World War II. This program not only demonstrated the US's goodwill to former adversaries like Germany and Italy, but also helped strengthen political alliances during the Cold War. After the Cold War, diplomacy gained even more importance in the new international order. With the merging of new states and new powers, the roles of diplomacy and communication became even more pronounced. The velvet revolution in the former Czechoslovakia was another great victory, using diplomatic solutions to resolve interstate issues. When in 1989 the former Czechoslovakia faced domestic upheaval about the independence of Slovakia, diplomacy was able to resolve the conflict without bloodshed. As a result, Czechoslovakia separated into two sovereign nations without any force being used. Finally, a more recent successful example of using diplomatic instruments is former President Clinton's visit to North Korea in 2009. His goal was to return American hostages to the US, using only his personal political influence to avoid any confrontation between

North Korea and the US. This example shows the diplomatic power of one uniquely quali-fied and well-known person. The successful return of the American journalists was also a great diplomatic move as the State Department was only remotely involved in the exchange; the incident did not provoke the official channels of the two countries, which did not have diplomatic relations at the time.

As the above examples demonstrated, diplomacy manifests itself through many dif-ferent tools, including official negotiations and cultural exchanges. Within these cultural exchanges, sport can play an important role because of its universal popularity and homo-geneous character (i.e., international rules and federations; Jackson & Haigh, 2008). To provide the reader with a stronger understanding of the traditional and the new applications of diplomacy, we start our chapter with a review of diplomacy in general, after which we will review the development of the theory of *soft power*. Soft power is a construct more recently introduced by political scholars; we will review the concept in more depth, as sport falls under this category. Finally, we will discuss the various objectives that governments could achieve through the use of sports.

DIPLOMACY

Modern diplomacy can be traced back to the 5th century's Italian city-states. The goal of diplomacy was to establish representation and create a communication channel between the monarch and the city-states. Since that period, communication channels have been domi-nated by the Western European languages, first French, and later, English. Today, modern technology allows for instant translation during international meetings. Once nation states became the dominant political entities in the world, the Westphalian notion of sovereign states (the principal in international law that sovereignty resides with each nation state) added to the importance of using diplomacy. Sovereignty became a symbol of equality among states, which used diplomacy to communicate among equal sovereign states.

Diplomacy is "the management of international relations by negotiation; the method by which these relations are adjusted by ambassadors and envoys; the business or art of the diplomatist" (Nicolson, 1964, p 4-5). A more current, shorter definition allows for a more ambiguous view on diplomacy: "the dialogue between states" (Watson, 1991, p. xii). This latter definition does not define the agents within the diplomacy process, nor does it acknowledge the role of nongovernmental agencies. Diplomacy is therefore the main instru-ment to implement national foreign policy during peace and is also a tool that can be used to communicate during conflict. The main features of diplomacy have been communica-tion and representation. Diplomacy has long been established as the first step to avoid or resolve conflicts. In addition, it helps with negotiations; protects the citizens and other interests abroad; promotes economic, social, cultural, and scientific exchanges between states; and manages foreign policy decisions. Diplomacy traditionally involves government-to-government contact, but there are other channels of communicating national interest and influencing other countries. After the official diplomatic recognition between states, the dialogue usually continues through other channels of diplomacy, such as educational exchange programs, concerts, or other cultural events.

Because of technological advances that have led to cheap and easy transportation and communication, the world is increasingly interconnected and many new tools are now available for diplomats. Bilateral negotiations and summit meetings have been the traditional approaches to resolving international issues, but in the 20th century, new diplomatic communications tools have emerged, such as public diplomacy (Cull, 2008), cultural diplomacy (Arnd, 2005), and cyberdiplomacy (Potter, 2002). Since the beginning of the 20th century, how diplomacy is conducted and who the actors are have changed significantly. From the traditional way of diplomats communicating their state's preferences at summits or at multilateral negotiations, modern diplomacy has moved to operating through many new channels and actors. The government may not even participate in these exchanges, but instead an athlete, artist, or scientist can represent the interests of the state at various events.

Multilateral institutions like the United Nations or the International Olympic Committee, global firms like Apple or Nike, and individuals such as famous athletes or actors can now represent their states. This new type of diplomatic representation can have both positive and negative outcomes. While it gives governments another outlet to work through, it could also prioritize the corporate interests of a nation over its political interests when these two conflict. In addition, the traditional venue of diplomacy has also moved towards economic or cultural forums or international sports events such as the Olympics. While there is still some scholarly disagreement about these new types of diplomatic actors and venues, the shift from traditional ways must be noted (Pigman, 2010).

While sovereignty has remained key in international negotiations and diplomatic recognitions, it no longer implies that only official diplomats can serve as representatives of a nation's interest and culture (Pigman, 2010). Indeed, in the 21st century more nonstate actors such as individuals, teams, and even companies can function as representatives of their nation. This is another reason why today even sports teams or individuals can become the messengers of their nation's diplomatic messages. Famous artists or athletes can act as bridges between nations and can help to resolve national issues via cultural and sport diplomacy. These lesser known diplomatic instruments serve as great examples of how governments can influence other states indirectly. While the athletes usually do not directly participate in the negotiations, the athletic event serves as a great venue for heads of state and diplomats to meet and discuss issues. This influence based on the attraction of countries is also called *soft power*.

HARD POWER AND SOFT POWER

Power remains one of the key concepts in international relations (Machiavelli, 1532/2010 Morgenthau, 1948; Deutsch, 1967; Kissinger, 1994). For many years Realist and Neorealist scholars viewed interstate relations in terms of states seeking power and wanting to dominate other states. In this conceptualization, international politics is a struggle for power

(Morgenthau, 1948), tends to only consider power in terms of capability (land, military, wealth, etc.), and is most commonly applied to armed conflicts. While power has been broadly defined as the ability to influence (Dahl, 1957; Morgenthau, 1973; Deutsch, 1967), Nye (1990) later separated power into the categories of *hard power* and *soft power*. Today, hard power usually refers to military interventions or economic payments or sanctions. This interpretation of power, however, fails to address the more subtle aspects of power, such as the influence of culture in general or sport events in particular, in which states can use their cultural prowess to affect changes in other nations. Nye's (1990) concept of soft power thus recognizes the way in which power is exercised through democratic values, human rights, and opportunities, and other seductive values (Nye, 1990, 2004a).

The US's strength in soft power has often been the focus of soft power research, but studying other applications of soft power, such as President Putin's hosting of the Sochi Olympics or Brazil's organization of the soccer World Cup, are less obvious research topics (see "From Diplomatic Dwarf to Gulliver Unbound: Brazil and the Use of Sports Mega-Events" and "Putin and the 2014 Winter Olympics: Russia's Authoritarian Sports Diplomacy" in this book). For Nye, soft power is a strong shaper of foreign public opinion and is a cheaper option than force. Nye's definition of the sources of soft power includes culture, political values, and foreign policy (Nye, 2004a). As such, sport may play an important role as a form of soft power, and therefore, it is important to study and understand the range of contexts within which it has been most effective.

In today's increasingly interconnected international system, countries try to utilize their diplomatic assets to their fullest. Sport can play an important role in this process, because of its universal popularity and its ability to serve as common ground between nations. It allows hosts and guests to converse about an issue they both have knowledge of and can feel comfortable to disagree on, because of its nonsensitive nature (Chalip, 2006). The popularity of world-class sport events can enable the initiation of multilateral diplomacy. In terms of foreign policy tools, sport also serves as an instrument to wield soft power. As noted earlier, this chapter will shed light on the role that sport can play and will highlight both successful and unsuccessful examples.

SPORT DIPLOMACY

International sporting events continue to mediate estrangement among people and their governments by promoting intercultural understanding and cooperation. Using the Olympics to improve a country's image abroad or to better the relationship between countries has been a diplomatic tool since the Olympics in ancient Greece (Pigman, 2010). Sporting events are useful because both the spectators (people) and their governments (elite politicians) can be reached through their love of sport. As a consequence, international sporting events can also improve relations both bilaterally and multilaterally (Chehabi, 2001).

During the Cold War, bilateral sporting events were used repeatedly to increase communication among hostile countries. Ping-pong diplomacy, for instance, between China and the United States allowed two nations in the middle of the Cold War to restart dialogue in a politically divided environment. President Nixon's diplomatic move opened up relations with China, which resulted in an improved bilateral relationship between the two nations in the decades to come. Cricket diplomacy between India and Pakistan offered another illustration of successful sport diplomacy. Following the Soviet invasion of Afghanistan in 1987, General Zia ul-Haq, Pakistan's president at the time, attended a test cricket match between India and Pakistan in Jaipur—a visit that apparently helped cool a flare-up in tensions caused by Soviet pressure on India. Furthermore, in 2004 after a break of fifteen years, India toured Pakistan in the wake of diplomatic initiatives to bury half a century of mutual hostility. Both sides relaxed their tough visa regulations for each other, allowing thousands of fans to travel across the border.

Yet, sport can also worsen the relationship between nations, as the example of El Salvador and Honduras shows. The poor relationship between the two nations was caused by large numbers of migrants from El Salvador, who moved to Honduras in search of a better life. This poor relationship was further exacerbated by the three World Cup qualifying matches these two nations had to play against each other in the month of June in 1969. The same day that the third and final game was played between the two nations, El Salvador severed all diplomatic ties with Honduras and started bombing their neighboring nation. Ever since then, this war has been referred to as La Guerra del Futbol—the Soccer War. While in the past bilateral sport diplomacy played an important role in bringing two countries to the negotiating table, this chapter focuses on the multilateral aspect of sport diplomacy by looking into various government initiatives. The examples in this chapter illustrate different levels of success using *multilateral sport diplomacy.*

In terms of sport diplomacy, the fact that international organizations serve as the main organizers of events also creates a diplomatically comfortable situation in which a third-party civil organization can serve as a neutral host and mediator between parties. Some of the most prominent international sports organization are the International Olympic Committee (IOC), which organizes the modern Olympic Games; Fédération Internationale de Football (FIFA), which organizes the largest, most well known global sport event, the Soccer World Cup; and International Tennis Federation (ITF), which includes 205 national tennis federations. By organizing events, as well as sanctioning and facilitating the competitions, these organizations can be both causes of cultural alienation and mediators of cooperation (Chalip, 2006). Stated differently, international sporting events can mediate conflicts between nations but only when organized and delivered under the right circumstances. It has been noted in both international relations and sport diplomacy scholarship that international institutions can serve as vehicles for sharing norms among nations, which can facilitate cooperation but also can cause tension among nations (Risse-Kappen, 1995; Axelrod & Keohane, 1985).

The role of international sport events has recently become even more complicated as it is now a very lucrative global business. Through sponsors, government and private contracts, and tourism, these events can earn lots of money for both the government and for

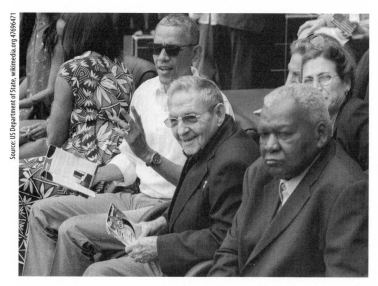

Source: US Department of State, wikimedia.org 47696471

U.S. President Barack Obama sits with Cuban President Raul Castro at the Estadio Lationamericano in Havana, Cuba, on March 22, 2016, for an exhibition game between the Cuban National Baseball Team and the Tampa Bay Rays.

private businesses. The following examples will illustrate how new diplomatic actors and venues can play important roles in conducting diplomacy. The examples will also illustrate some of the successful and failed practices of multilateral diplomacy through sports events.

SUCCESSFUL AND UNSUCCESSFUL SPORT DIPLOMACY STRATEGIES AND OUTCOMES

1. Sport provides an unofficial reason and location for international leaders to meet and begin a dialogue.

The potential diplomatic contributions of international sport events can be manifold. They can serve as a general outreach to the international community or strengthen the relations between two specific countries, one being the host (see "Sport for Hope in Haiti: Disaster Diplomacy or Disaster Capitalism," "Sport as a Political Strategy in North-South Korean Relations," and "Wrestling with Diplomacy: The US and Iran" in this book). Using the general popularity of sports, athletic events can be great excuses for unofficial meetings for leaders, and mega sports events can allow for large-scale diplomacy where a multitude of political leaders could meet. There are plenty of official meetings and summits for diplomats and heads of state, but few of them are as desirable and entertaining as sport events—nor do they receive as much media attention. While enjoying the performances of the elite athletes, including the ones from their own nations, many heads of state often use the opportunity to engage other parties in unofficial discussions about issues.

While mega sport events provide good venues for multilateral meetings, sometimes heads of state need an event that is specifically designed to resolve issues between two states. Ping-pong diplomacy was a great example of using a sport event to initiate political dialogue between two countries on opposite sides during the Cold War, as Nixon did by visiting China in 1972. Attending a bilateral sport event helps two countries' representatives work out their issues while enjoying the competition. In 1972, Nixon's decision to visit ended the long U.S. ostracism of China and was both a major event in modern diplomacy and a smart geostrategic move. It increased external pressure on the Soviet Union, facilitated the U.S. exit from the Vietnam conflict, and laid the foundation for subsequent Sino-American cooperation (Kissinger, 1994). South Korea provides another example of using a mega sport event as a successful tool in their international relations. They used the 1988 Summer Olympics in Seoul successfully as a tool to improve their relationships with the (then) USSR and Eastern European nations, and were successfully able to prevent these nations from boycotting the Olympics in support of North Korea.

Nevertheless, these meeting spaces should not be seen as exclusively positive, because such events can also legitimize a regime when an opposite response is warranted. The Berlin Olympics in 1936 offers a great example of this. Even though Germany won the bid for the Olympic Games two years before Hitler came to power, during a tense international period just before WWII, this multinational sporting event was used as political propaganda for the German Reich and an unofficial meeting place to talk about alignment in case of potential war. More recently, the Dutch royal family and Prime Minister came under strong criticism in 2014 for attending the Sochi Winter Olympics opening ceremony, while other foreign heads of state stayed at home in protest of the civil right violations against the LGBT community in Russia (Pinedo & Versteegh, 2014). The Dutch media perceived the delegation as legitimizing the Russian state, and their criticism highlights the scrutiny that can be placed on politicians to attend certain events and refrain from attending others.

2. Sport provides insight into the host country and educates others about it.
Many people, not just heads of state, want to enjoy large sport events and are proud of hosting them. Since 1936, when the Summer Games were first broadcast to 41 countries, hosting nations take great pride in beautifying their countries to project a positive image, and with the development of technology, billions of people can watch these sporting events on television or using various devices. This view of the competitions also provides information about the host cities, such as infrastructure, tourist attractions, and culture. In 1936, not only did the Games provide a meeting place for European and other leaders to discuss their political alignment, but the world saw the political ideology and domestic politics of Germany through the kind of state-controlled propaganda now often associated with mega sport events.

Today, billions of people can see into a host nation's domestic politics and political ideology. Mega-events such as the Olympics are witnessed around the world, not just broadcast on the official TV stations but also disseminated via YouTube and other social media outlets. Educating people about a nation's beautiful scenery and resources can benefit host nations in many ways, encouraging tourism, foreign-directed investment, and foreign students. Spreading the political ideology of the hosting government can influence both the foreign public and the leaders; as the example of the 1936 Nazi Olympics illustrates, these sport events can be used to mislead an international audience about the intentions of a particular regime.

While sport events can inform people around the world about the positives of a destination, they can also inform people of the negatives, as states are seldom able to entirely control the media exposure around the event (Giffard & Rivenburgh, 2000). Protest groups have understood the power of these events to convey their message to the media, and many have turned media attention to the negative aspects of the host nation, such as environmental issues (e.g., smog), human rights issues, health standards, high rates of HIV virus carriers, or specific problems such as the domestic dispute with Tibet in the lead-up to the Beijing Olympics, the economic inequality in South Africa, and the water pollution and home evictions in Brazil. Additionally, the opportunity to host these mega-events is no longer uncontested, and the exorbitant costs and the many corruption charges against federations such as FIFA and the IOC have made people around the world very critical. As a result, nations need to think carefully about how to present themselves through the international media and understand that these events spotlight a nation in ways that can be both negative and positive.

3. Using sport to bridge cultural and linguistic differences among nations through sports. Sporting events have another special feature. Because most people who watch a competition already know the rules, the events bridge cultural and linguistic gulfs that may exist between the hosting nation and the spectators. It does not matter if the hosting nation is Russia, China, or Brazil, millions of sport fans are cheering for their favorite athletes despite the language used in the broadcast. There are numerous ways to use the connecting effect of sport events, and they can also be used on a much smaller scale for diplomatic purposes. Sports teams, as well as individual athletes, can be used to educate people about countries and also promote mutual understanding of different cultures.

A recent example of a head of state deliberately using a sport event to bring two different nations together is President Obama's 2016 visit to Cuba. During his trip, the U.S. President not only reconnected the two nations diplomatically, but by attending a baseball game, he also took a significant step towards bridging the ideological and political differences between Cuba and the U.S, reminding the Cubans of a shared passion for the game of baseball. As noted earlier, watching a sport event, such as a baseball game, bridges linguistic, cultural, and political differences between nations, and in the case of Cuba and the US, it pointed to the common interest of two presidents and their nations.

4. Sport can be used to create a platform for new legislation or trade agreements. Mega sport events also provide a good illustration of the role sport can play in regards to legislation or trade agreements. International federations, most notably FIFA and the IOC, have certain guarantees associated with hosting their events and require governmental approval. The most influential guarantee related to diplomacy is the visa requirement that these organizations impose on their hosts. In order to prevent hosts from excluding particular nations from their events (i.e., China and Taiwan, United States and Iran, etc.), the host nation is not allowed to withhold a visa from anyone who is associated with the event. To illustrate, when the Netherlands bid for the 2018 FIFA World Cup, they had to put the following guarantee in their bid:

The Netherlands, represented by its Government, represents, warrants, ensures and guarantees to FIFA for the purposes of entry into and exit from the Netherlands, and for a period commencing on the date of this Guarantee and ending on [31 December 2018 /31 December 2022], that entry visas and exit permits shall be issued unconditionally and without any restriction and, where issuance of formal visas or permits is not required, the right to entry to and exit from the Netherlands, shall be granted unconditionally and without any restriction, and regardless of nationality, race or creed, to... [followed by a long list of all FIFA stakeholders, including FIFA employees, sponsors, broadcasters, athletes and spectators]. (Heere, 2012)

When Korea and Japan were asked to co-host the 2002 FIFA World Cup, the two nations used the event to start a dialogue and improve on their historically problematic relationship. However, the organization of the event itself became symbolic of the problematic relationship between the two nations, and the two nations fought openly about the name of the tournament, the mascot, and the location of the important matches (opening match, semifinals, and final). Still, the event did allow for a stronger bilateral relationship between the two nations (Heere et al., 2012). The most notable changes were caused by bilateral agreements between the two nations: visa regulations for visitors from the other nation were loosened up and different economic forums and symposia were held in the years surrounding the World Cup. In 2004, the Korean Overseas Information system reported that the event had initiated increased political dialogue between South Korea and Japan as a direct consequence of joint-hosting the event (Heere et al., 2012).

Sport mega-events are also associated with a strong increase in trade agreements between the host and the rest of the world. Rose and Spiegel (2011) argued that hosting a mega-event such as the Olympics signals to the rest of the world that the nation is "open for business," and they report export and import increases in nations that have hosted the Games, often related to the trade agreements that nations are able to make before, during, and directly after the event.

5. Sport can be used to create awareness for the international relationship through sport ambassadors.

As we mentioned earlier, sports teams, events, and even individual athletes can become sports ambassadors and can provide a face to the nation. A benefit of sport events and individual athletes over official diplomats and politicians is that the negotiations can be seen less as government directed and more as free and spontaneous. In an international environment when governments face criticism for practicing too much control, allowing less restricted forms of diplomacy to occur can be refreshing and welcomed. Also, including the individuals as ambassadors who are not otherwise affiliated with their governments and can speak through their athletic achievements can also bring a fresh start to a relationship between nations that may have previously been complicated by problems and distrust. Whereas some people instantly distrust politicians, athletes are generally well-liked and admired, and can provide cultural empathy among people. They provide a friendly and positive face to a nation. Watching the performance of world-class athletes has been one of the favorite activities of political leaders as well as most ordinary people.

Many former athletes have chosen political careers after their athletic careers have ended, and have used their celebrity to create new relations. For instance, after his basketball career, Bill Bradley became a U.S. senator and in 1992 was a sponsor of a bill called the Freedom Support Act that allowed for exchanges between the Soviet Union and the United States (Cox, 2007). Former athletes such as Pele, George Weah, and Manny Pacquiao all have become politicians in their own nations to shape domestic and foreign policies. International organizations such as the United Nations have also understood the power of athletes to build international relationships and have structured ambassador programs in which many athletes participate: Muhammed Ali, Carl Lewis, Maria Sharapova, Marta, Didier Drogba, and the list goes on (www.un.org).

Sport ambassadors do not necessarily have to be famous athletes. One great example of public diplomacy is the U.S. Department of State's Bureau of Educational and Cultural Affairs (BECA); see "CultureConnect and the U.S. Department of State: A Gateway to the Future of Sport Diplomacy." This office has many programs, one of which is SportsUnited, which sends American athletes on international cultural exchange missions and brings foreign athletes to the US for clinics and exhibition games. Secretary of State Hillary Clinton has said,

> Actually, our sport's exchanges are the most popular exchanges we do. And when I go to other countries around the world and we talk about what kind of exchanges that people are looking for, very often a leader will say, how about a sports exchange? (Clinton, 2011)

Along with art and music, sports are one of those areas of human commonalities that require little interpretation. SportsUnited describes the program as,

> an international sports programming initiative designed to help start a dialogue at the grassroots level with non-elite young people. The programs aid youth in discovering how success in athletics can be translated into the development of life skills and achievement in the classroom. (Clinton, 2011)

Additionally, professional athletes can bridge cultural differences because they enjoy worldwide admiration. Athletes such as Yao Ming (China), Vlade Divac (Yugoslavia/Serbia), George Weah (Liberia), and Kathy Freeman (Aboriginal population Australia) have put a face to a nation or an ethnic group that people knew little about, thereby providing knowledge and understanding to those outside their particular culture.

Sport can also do the opposite, and sport teams and athletes can serve a national propaganda machine meant to support a negative narrative. Both the victories of chess grandmaster Bobby Fischer (over Boris Spassky in 1972) and the U.S. hockey team (over the Soviet Union in 1980) were used to support the Cold War narrative and demonstrate U.S. superiority over the Soviet Union. In the late 1980s, the rivalry between the Netherlands and Germany in football was highlighted by two incidents that worsened the relationship between the two nations, and revived (undeservedly) an anti-Germany sentiment in the Netherlands. First, in 1988, Ronald Koeman used the shirt of German player Olaf Thon (football players often swap jerseys after the match as a token of mutual appreciation) to make an offensive gesture, and two years later, a spat between Frank Rijkaard and Rudi Voller at the 1990 World Cup led to the expulsion of both players from the field. These are examples in which athletes actually play a negative role in emphasizing cultural differences and historical divides, negatively affecting the bilateral relationship between the two nations (Altijd weer dat shirt van Olaf Thon, 2008). In that light, the invitation of Dennis Rodman (former NBA player) by North Korea is an interesting case, an instructive example of both the power of elite athletes and also the complexity of having a nondiplomat play a diplomatic role. The fact that the leader of North Korea, Kim Jong-Un, was willing to allow an American TV crew into his country and into his life in 2013 is the result of basketball's popularity and the fact the young leader is a huge fan of NBA basketball and Dennis Rodman. As there was no official diplomatic relationship between the US and North Korea at the time, letting an American athlete and his TV crew film North Korea and provide an insight into this country was a great diplomatic contribution. However, as we later learned, having a diplomatically untrained athlete serve as the eye of the US and the West is definitely not without limitations. As U.S. State Department officials learned after Rodman's trip, while the athlete was able to satisfy Kim Jong-Un's desire to play basketball with a superstar, he did not have the necessary diplomatic sophistication and patience a true sport ambassador needs to successfully conduct both the preparation and the aftermath of such events.

Another creative and effective way of using individual athletes as sport ambassadors is the US's approach to allowing the recruitment of the best foreign athletes to play collegiate sports in the US. Providing sports grants and sports scholarships for foreign athletes to study in American colleges are great examples of encouraging cultural exchanges using both the platform of sports and cultures. There are over 2,000 universities in the US, many of which offer scholarships for athletes. Because the coaches are pressured to have the most competitive teams, they often recruit athletes from abroad with athletic scholarships. These elite athletes not only bring victory for their U.S. college teams, but also bring their own culture. During a typical four-year term, similar to an exchange program, foreign athletes become sport ambassadors to their countries as they share their cultures with teammates and other students. At the same time, the foreign athlete also lives in the US, which serves as a great educational and cultural experience.

6. Sport events can be used to create a legacy for the host country, improving its image in the world.

Creating a legacy is one of the most commonly used reasons for hosting a large sport event. For countries that are trying to improve their image abroad, organizing a successfully run sport event is a great opportunity to showcase not only the firm institutional and organizational grounds of the state, but also to allow the visitors and spectators to see the cultural and geographic beauty of the host nation. One of the oldest sport events in the world is the Tour de France, an annual sport cycling race that showcases the nation to the world every year. Because the sport is best viewed from the air, the Tour de France makes extensive use of helicopters, which showcase not only the cyclists, but also provide views of the beautiful French landscapes, and historic towns and castles, and the event has played an important role in the image-building process of France around the world (Heere et al., 2015).

Similarly, mega sport events, such as the Olympics and the FIFA World Cup, have often been used to show the progress a developing nation has been making and can change the somewhat antiquated views that Western viewers, in particular, have of the nation. The Summer Olympics in 1964 in Tokyo might have been the first example of this tradition, but other organizers, such as Mexico City (1968 Summer Olympics and 1970 FIFA World Cup), Seoul (1988 Summer Olympics), Barcelona (1992 Summer Olympics), Beijing (2008 Summer Olympics), and South Africa (2010 FIFA World Cup) were all used to show their host city or nation as modern, "Westernized" destinations with universally accepted values.

These prestigious events are also seen as ways for a nation to show their hard power, which might not necessarily improve the image of the nation around the world but simply shows that they are a nation to be reckoned with. This use of sport events to show a nation's power has been a long-time tradition, perhaps starting as early as 1934, when Mussolini used the FIFA World Cup to show Italy's superiority, a strategy repeated two years later by Hitler at the 1936 Summer Olympics. Since then, nations such as the United Kingdom (1948 Summer Olympics), Argentina (1978 FIFA World Cup), China (2008 Summer Olympics), United States (Summer Olympics 1984, Winter Olympics of 1980 and 2002), and Russia (Summer Olympics of 1980 and Winter Olympics of 2014) have all used these events to show their power to the rest of the world.

The most recent example of such ambitions, the Sochi Winter Olympic Games showed the intricacies associated with the attempt to use mega-events as tools to show off both hard and soft power. The Sochi event showed the world that even in times of international tensions and doubts about Russia's foreign policy goals, President Putin could use the event to implement foreign policy through multiple channels (Simonyi & Trunkos, 2014). To some extent, the event was a success for Russia. The main issue during the Sochi Olympics was security. President Putin had to ensure that nothing interrupted the safety of spectators and athletes at the event despite the threat of domestic ethnic conflicts, and he did so successfully. By allowing the visitors to better understand Russia through the sports events, President Putin created a window into what he thought was a perfectly controlled image of Russia and one that his own constituency in Russia was very supportive of. Also, the success of Russian athletes supported the narrative of the Russian resurrection as a world power (see "Putin and the 2014 Winter Olympics: Russia's Authoritarian Sports Diplomacy").

Nevertheless, despite the successes, Sochi came at a price for Russia. As they had done at other events, global media emphasized the poor human rights for the LGBT community in Russia and the environmental disaster that Sochi might produce for the region; the exorbitant costs of the event showcased how little power Putin has over the corporate elites in his nation. Moreover, any goodwill that Sochi might have built up around the world was destroyed a year later, when Russia decided to invade the Crimean Peninsula and support the pro-Russia faction in the Ukraine.

7. Sport can be used to provide legitimacy for a new nation.
As noted in the earlier sections, international sport events attract the attention of millions of people, including sport fans and political leaders. This global stage can be used to achieve the previously listed outcomes, but it can also be used as a platform for a symbolic fight for a country's political independence. For instance, international sport federations often offer the opportunity for territories that have the ambition to become independent nation-states and compete under a flag that might not actually represent the current sovereign nation. For instance, there has been political tension between the People's Republic of China and Taiwan for many years. Taiwan has been fighting for its political independence from China. As a result of political negotiations and the IOC's decision in 1980, the athletic teams of Taiwan are now allowed to compete under the Chinese Taipei flag, which is separate from the Chinese flag. This solution has been accepted for numerous international sport events such as the Olympic Games, the World Baseball Classic and the FIFA World Cup. This is not only a political victory for Taiwan but it also allows Taiwanese athletes to express their feelings about independence and it provides opportunities for the athletes to compete against China in the games. Similarly, in the years after World War II, Israel actively used sport in their quest for international recognition of their nation (Galily & Ben-Porat, 2009).

Even if a particular quest is unsuccessful, sport can still shed light upon the occupation of one nation by another. The Hungary versus USSR water polo game at the 1956 Melbourne Olympics was a good example of this. The Hungarians rebelled against the oppression of the Soviet Union in October of 1956 but were defeated in a bloody fight. Later in the year, the Hungarian national team ended up playing against the Soviet team in the Olympic Games and the Hungarians won. While the sport victory of the Hungarian team did not lead to better treatment of the Hungarians at home, it gained the sympathy of millions of sport fans after the bloody events of the revolution.

CONCLUSION

We attempted in this chapter to outline different ways governments can use sport as an international policy tool. Following Chalip (2006), we acknowledge that sport can have both a negative and positive effect on society, and we attempted to showcase some of the best and worst examples of how sport has been used by political regimes. Sport events, athletes, and teams can provide a face to a nation and a useful instrument to exert their soft power and showcase their hard power to the world, but only if they are used and leveraged correctly. In today's complicated and fast-paced, technology-driven world, every opportunity to promote a country's positive image abroad must be taken, and politicians are well served with the knowledge of how to use sport to fit their purposes. Placing the spotlight on a nation through sports can be advantageous and provide worldwide attention to positive changes. Seoul used the Summer Olympics to improve their relationships with the Soviet Union and the nations in their hemisphere. Barcelona used the Summer Olympics to showcase that they were no longer burdened by the heritage of Franco and were an attractive tourist destination in Europe. However, events could also lead to an emphasis on larger domestic issues challenging a nation. A fascinating example was provided by Athens that, because of its historic ties to the Olympics, was seen as a perfect host to the event. However, in the lead-up, global media often emphasized the lack of progress in building the required infrastructure. The high costs of organizing the event also placed an economic burden on the nation that contributed to its economic collapse a decade later (Heere, 2012). Sport plays an enormous role in our daily lives and, similar to other cultural global phenomena such as popular music, food, and dance, sport entails a universal language that everyone speaks. As Nelson Mandela once stated, "Sport has the power to change the world, to inspire and to unite people in a way that very little else can" (Korr & Close, 2008). Yet that power is not a given and only manifests itself when sport managers and politicians understand how to leverage sport correctly to achieve the objectives associated with it in the first place.

DISCUSSION QUESTIONS

1. How can states leverage international sport events to strengthen their international relations?
2. What is soft power and how is sport diplomacy connected to it?
3. What are the most common strategic objectives when relying on sport diplomacy?
4. Are these strategic objectives always achieved? List some of the successful and unsuccessful examples.
5. Based on this chapter, please explain which strategic outcomes Brazil wished to achieve with the summer Olympic Games. What issues did they have to overcome and how did they use the Olympics to achieve them?

REFERENCES

Altijd weer dat shirt van Olaf Thon: De Duitsers en het EK'88. (9 Juni, 2008). Het Duitsland Instituut. Retrieved from https://duitslandinstituut.nl/artikel/3267/altijd-weer-dat-shirt-van-olaf-thon
Arndt, R. T. (2005). *The first resort of kings: American cultural diplomacy in the twentieth century.* Washington, DC: Potomac Books, Inc.
Axelrod, R., & Keohane, R. O. (1985). Achieving cooperation under anarchy: Strategies and institutions. *World Politics, 38*(1), 226-254.

Bachrach, P., & Baratz, M. S. (1963). Decisions and nondecisions: An analytical framework. *American Political Science Review, 57,* 632-642.

Bayne, N., & Woolcock, S. (Eds.). (2011). *The new economic diplomacy: Decision-making and negotiation in international economic relations.* Surrey, UK: Ashgate Publishing, Ltd.

Center for Strategic and International Studies Commission on Smart Power: Hearings before the Foreign Relations Committee, Senate, 110th Cong. (2008, April 24). (Testimony of J. S. Nye, Jr. & R. L. Armitage).

Chalip, L. (2006). Toward a distinctive sport management discipline. *Journal of Sport Management, 20,* 1-21.

Chehabi, H. E. (2001). Sport diplomacy between the United States and Iran. *Diplomacy and Statecraft, 12,* 89-106.

Clinton. H. R. (2011, June 6) *Remarks on the launching of the women's World Cup initiative.* Speech presented in the Benjamin Franklin Room. Washington, DC.

Cox, E. (September 7, 2007). New faces from abroad: Exchange students bring different cultural perspectives to gorge. *The Dalles Chronicle.* Retrieved from http://nl.newsbank.com/nl-search/we/Archives?p_action=doc&p_docid=11BA13F4B02A94E8&p_docnum=8

Cull, N. J. (2008). Public diplomacy: Taxonomies and histories. *The Annals of the American Academy of Political and Social Science, 616,* 31-54.

Dahl, R. A. (1957). The concept of power. *Behavioral Science, 2,* 201–215.

Deutsch, K. W. (1967). On the concepts of politics and power. *Journal of International Affairs, 21,* 232-241.

Galily, Y., & Ben-Porat, A. (2009). *Sport, politics and society in the land of Israel: Past and present.* New York, NY: Routledge.

Giffard, C. A., & Rivenburgh, N. K. (2000). News agencies, national images, and global media events. *Journalism & Mass Communication, 77,* 8-21.

Gilboa, E. (2008). Searching for a theory of public diplomacy. *The Annals of the American Academy of Political and Social Science, 616,* 55-77.

Goodwill ambassadors. (n.d.). The United Nations. Retrieved from http://www.un.org/wcm/content/site/sport/home/unplayers/goodwillambassadors on December 8th, 2015

Heere, B. (2015). *Het effect van de Tour de France organisatie op het imago van Utrecht in de wereld.* (Report for the city of Utrecht.) Columbia, SC: Pictura Magna.

Heere, B. (2012). *Het Olympisch Speeltje.* Amsterdam, Netherlands: Atlas-Contact.

Heere, B., Kim, C., Yoshida, M., Nakamura, H., Ogura, T., Chung, K. S., & Lim, S. Y. (2012). The impact of World Cup 2002 on the bilateral relationship between South Korea and Japan. *Journal of Sport Management, 26,* 127-142.

Jackson, S. J., & Haigh, S. (2008). Between and beyond politics: Sport and foreign policy in a globalising world. *Sport in Society, 11,* 349-358.

Keohane, R. O. and J. S. Nye, Jr. (2001). *Power and interdependence* (3rd ed). New York, NY: Longman.

Kissinger, H. (1994). *Diplomacy.* New York, NY: Simon & Schuster Paperbacks.

Korr, C., & Close, M. (2008). *More than just a game.* London, UK: Harper Collins.

Lukes, S. (1974). *Power: A radical view* (2nd ed). London, UK: Palgrave Macmillan.

Machiavelli, N. (1532/2010). *The Prince.* Chicago, IL: University of Chicago Press.

Morgenthau, H. (1948). *Politics among nations: The struggle for power and peace.* New York, NY: Alfred A Knopf.

Nicolson, Sir H. (1964). *Diplomacy* (3rd ed.) New York: Oxford University Press.

Nye, J. S., Jr. (1990). *Bound to lead: The changing nature of American power.* New York, NY: Basic Books.

Nye, J. S., Jr. (2002). Limits of American power. *Political Science Quarterly, 11*(4), 554.

Nye, J. S., Jr. (2004a). *Soft power: The means to success in world politics.* New York, NY: Public Affairs.

Nye, J. S., Jr. (2004b). *Soft Power and American Foreign Policy*. Political Science Quarterly, 119, 255-270.

Nye, J. S., Jr. (2011). *The future of power*. New York, NY. Public Affairs.

Pigman, G. A. (2010). *Contemporary diplomacy. Representation and communication in a globalized world*. Cambridge, UK: Polity.

Pinedo, D., & Versteegh, K. (January 15th, 2014). Debat Sotsji maakt positive koning Willem-Alexander kwetsbaar. NRC Handelsblad. Retrieved from http://www.nrc.nl/nieuws/2014/01/15/debat-sotsji-maakt-positie-koning-willem-alexander-kwetsbaar on December 8th, 2015/

Potter, E. H. (2002). *Cyber-diplomacy: Managing foreign policy in the twenty-first century*. Montreal and Kingston: McGill-Queen's University Press.

Risse-Kappen, T. (1995). *Bringing transnational relations back in: Non-state actors, domestic structures and international institutions* (Vol. 42). Cambridge, UK Cambridge University Press.

Rose, A. K., & Spiegel, M. M. (2011). Do mega sport events promote international trade? *SAIS Review of International Affairs, 31*, 77-85.

Simonyi, A., & Trunkos J. (2014). How Putin stole our smart power. *Huffington Post*. Retrieved from http://www.huffingtonpost.com/andras-simonyi/how-putin-stole-our-smart_b_5504985.html

Watson, A. (1991). *Diplomacy: The dialogue between states*. London: Routledge.

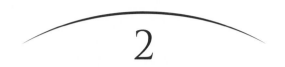

2

THE UNITED STATES GOVERNMENT'S ROLE IN SPORT DIPLOMACY

CARRIE LECROM · MELISSA FERRY

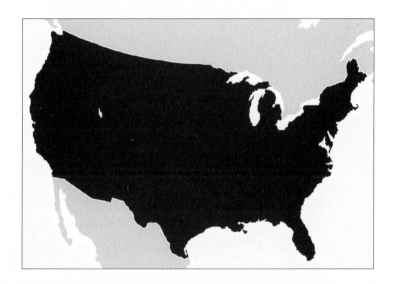

HISTORY

The United States government has engaged in sport diplomacy for decades. The 14 U.S. athletes who brought home 11 championships in the 1896 Olympic Games in Athens, Greece, marked an effort at expanding beyond our own borders to engage with foreign countries through sport. The Greeks, in founding the Olympics, viewed the games as a way to unify nations in spite of political differences (Goldberg, 2000). While not couched as a political endeavor, the Olympic Games and other international sport competitions (Pan Am Games, World Championships, Goodwill Games, Maccabi Games, Paralympic Games, etc.) have continued to be a strong form of diplomacy for the United States. For instance, the US continues to observe the Olympic Truce (a promise of peace during the Olympic Games) during each Olympic Games, as it has since 1896 (Sanders, 2011). The US made strong political statements during the 1960 and 1980 Olympic Games. Hosting the 1960 Olympics in Squaw Valley, California, the U.S. government refused to grant visas to athletes from East Germany. And in response to the Soviet Union's invasion of Afghanistan, the US boycotted the 1980 Olympic Games in Moscow, becoming one of 63 nations that refused to compete that year (Goldberg, 2000). These are but a few examples of ways the U.S. government has viewed sport as a diplomatic tool for decades.

During President Eisenhower's time in office, he sought to improve the physical fitness of Americans, hoping to boost the physical fitness of children and military draftees (Hunt, 2006). This changed notion of patriotic fitness was verbalized succinctly by Shane McCarthy, the executive director of the President's Council on Youth Fitness: "Perhaps as we consider the next Olympics, the theme should be not so much 'Win [in the 1960 games in] Rome' as 'Win at home'" (Hunt, 2006, p. 276). However, it was President Kennedy who initiated the presidential belief that the physical health of Americans was crucial for winning the Cold War (Hunt, 2006). In 1964 the Assistant Secretary of State for East Asian and Pacific Affairs suggested that media coverage of the Olympics in Tokyo could provide footage of friendly relations between American Olympians and individuals in Asia and Africa (Hunt, 2006). This seed spawned an effort to publicize the many ways the United States was cultivating better national images on behalf of particular countries through sport. This journey into sport diplomacy led to the Department of State's American Specialists program, which sent 57 sports specialists abroad during 1966, receiving positive international feedback and set the stage for a more encompassing program (Hunt, 2006).

However, a more politically direct, modern effort of sport diplomacy in the United States grew from April of 1971, when China invited the American ping-pong team to play a series of matches in mainland China. *Ping-pong diplomacy,* as it became known, is "the employment of international table tennis tournaments as a diplomatic tool to break the stalemate in relations among nations where the official diplomatic channels are absent or stalled" (Itoh, 2011, p. 3). At the time the American team was invited to visit China, the two countries were coming off several decades of hostile relations. Since the communist takeover of China in 1949, the United States had viewed the country as an enemy force. The US demonstrated its opposition to China by refusing to recognize the People's Republic of China (PRC) as the ruling government, disapproving of its communist reign, fighting on opposing sides through the Korean and Vietnam wars, and placing a trade embargo on the PRC (Itoh, 2011).

However, as the Vietnam war subsided, the iciness between the two countries began to recede. Incoming U.S. President Richard Nixon noted publicly his desire to broker peaceful relations between the two countries, stating at his 1969 Inaugural Address,

> The greatest honor history can bestow is the title of peacemaker. This honor
> now beckons America—the chance to help lead the world at last out of the

valley of turmoil onto that high ground of peace that man has dreamed of since the dawn of civilization. ("Address by Richard M. Nixon," 1969)

By 1971, little progress had been made despite Nixon's attempts at opening the lines of communication, making the invitation to the U.S. athletes that much more unexpected.

The ping-pong diplomacy trip in April 1971 marked the first time a group of Americans had been invited to China since the Communist takeover in 1949. Chinese Premier Chou En-lai, commenting on the series of matches, stated "never before in history has sport been used so effectively as a tool of international diplomacy" (DeVoss, 2002, p. 4). The Chinese hosts adopted a friendship-first-competition-second approach to the historic event, forging positive impressions in the minds of both sets of athletes. This positive encounter led to a covert visit by National Security Advisor Henry Kissinger to China in July of 1971, followed soon after by an official visit by President Nixon in 1972, the first U.S. President to visit the former communist country (Gerin, 2007; Itoh, 2011).

Following the successes of the American Specialists program in 1966, and ping-pong diplomacy in the '70s, over the next several decades, the US continued to utilize sport to develop international relationships (Hunt, 2006). Teams in nearly every organized sport (e.g., tennis, swimming, diving, track and field, basketball, soccer, volleyball, acrobatics, martial arts) made annual trips to China, and expanded these tours into other countries with whom the US was interested in developing stronger ties (Orlins, 2012). American wrestlers traveled to Iran in 1998 on a tournament invitation, paving the way for a peaceful meeting of the U.S. and Iranian soccer teams in the 1998 World Cup. Publicized as a grudge match by media, then U.S. President Bill Clinton recorded a pregame message discussing the opportunity for this match to end the estrangement between countries. The players competed with the highest levels of professionalism and integrity toward one another, and FIFA jointly awarded both nations the FIFA Fair Play Award for this performance (Chehabi, 2001; Goldberg, 2000; see "Wrestling with Diplomacy: The US and Iran" for details).

The US has also used sport as a diplomatic tool to make a statement. President Jimmy Carter decided to boycott the 1980 Moscow Olympic Games after the Soviet Union invaded Afghanistan. The Soviet Union followed suit in 1984, boycotting the Games that were held in Los Angeles (Goldberg, 2000). In addition, hoping to open up a dialogue that had stalled, the Baltimore Orioles traveled to Cuba in 1999 to play a friendly match; players returned with first-hand knowledge of the impact of the U.S. embargo on Cuba and an opportunity for conversations about the future of the relationship between countries (Goldberg, 2000). Despite efforts such as these, no other U.S. President after Jimmy Carter had a formal government-sponsored sport diplomacy program until George W. Bush (Gerin, 2007).

SPORTSUNITED

It was 43rd U.S. President George W. Bush who decided to elevate the credibility of the political strategy by formalizing it nearly 35 years after the successful ping-pong diplomacy initiative. In 2002, following the 9-11 terrorist attacks on the United States, the SportsUnited program was established to encourage interactions between youth in the United States and other countries through sport, focusing mainly on Muslim countries at the time. Shortly following, in 2006, President Bush created the United States' first public diplomacy envoy program, housed under the U.S Department of State's Bureau of Educational and Cultural Affairs (ECA), where it remains today. In establishing the envoy program, figure skater Michelle Kwan and baseball legend Cal Ripken Jr. were named as its inaugural representatives (Gerin, 2007). Kwan and Ripken traveled to China in 2007 to run clinics and programming for youth in several cities, with the ultimate goal of improving US-Chinese relations. During his Chinese visit Ripken commented,

> Sport in general has the ability to communicate to all people similar to what music does. It kind of goes across all lines, and I think baseball can resonate with people who use it to have fun and open up dialogues. (Gerin, 2007, p. 14)

(See "CultureConnect and the U.S. Department of State: A Gateway to the Future of Sport Diplomacy" for a case study.)

The SportsUnited program has grown into a strong and thriving branch of the U.S. State Department's Bureau of Educational and Cultural Affairs. ECA's stated mission is to "increase mutual understanding of the people of the United States and the people of other countries by means of educational and cultural exchange" ("About ECA," n.d.). Sport is a major vehicle for this, as evidenced by the growth and complexity of SportsUnited's people-to-people exchanges. The budget for these programs grew from approximately $600,000 in 2002 to over $5 million in 2007 (Walters, 2007), and has remained above $5 million annually since that time, demonstrating the U.S. government's continued commitment to diplomacy through sport.

As of 2016, SportsUnited thrives on four major prongs: a visitors program, an envoy program, a grant program, and a global sports mentoring program. Each program's unique components drive its success in achieving the overarching goals of the State Department and ECA.

Visitors Program

Through the Sports Visitors program, groups of foreign youth athletes, coaches, and administrators travel to the United States for two-week programs. The U.S.-based residencies cover topics such as nutrition, strength and conditioning, gender equality in sport, sport and disability, and team building, among other things ("Sports Envoys," n.d.). Delegations comprise non-elite athletes with the goal of developing cross-cultural understanding, building relationships, and developing skills and knowledge to take back to their home countries.

A look inside. Unwavering passion for their sports brought foreign athletes Fiorella Yriberry and Jesse Bernard to the United States for training through the SportsUnited Sports Visitors program, delivered through a cooperative agreement with the Center for Sport Management at George Mason University. Fiorella grew up surrounded by deep gender inequity in Bolivia, so was honored when she was selected to spend four weeks training, learning, and engaging with girls her age from around the world as part of the 2011 Women's World Cup program. Spending time in Washington, D.C., and New York City, she returned to Bolivia with best friends from Palestine and South Africa, as well as a new passion: empowering women in her community through soccer. Fellow athletes engaged in the SportsUnited initiative encouraged and supported her wish to create change in her home community. Once back in Bolivia, Fiorella quickly crafted an after-school soccer program for girls. She reflects that,

> the program is now running sustainably for more than three years, it does not only give young girls a chance to play the most fabulous game of all but also gives them educational session for ways in which they can improve their life conditions and opportunities as females (F. Yriberry, personal communication, December 4, 2015).

Having attended the SportsUnited program at just 16, Fiorella's mind-opening trip helped her to realize "that the most important thing... is knowing that I am a strong female able and capable of empowering my community to break away from gender roles and create equality" (F. Yriberry, personal communication, December 4, 2015).

In the Philippines, Jesse Bernard was already running a baseball and softball organization when he got the call in 2012 from SportsUnited, inviting him to Arizona. The Sports Visitors Philippine Baseball coaches training "was one of the highlights of my career" (J. Bernard, personal communication, December 2, 2015), learning new training techniques, updating teaching skills, and offering new innovations. The time stateside gave Jesse the

> opportunity to learn from the best coaches in America, see real games live, talk and pick the minds of highly respected personnel involved in the sport, and lastly, it gave me the opportunity to give back to the community back home by sharing what I learned during the training (J. Bernard, personal communication, December 2, 2015).

From his experience he wishes "other individuals from the Philippines will be given the same opportunity I had in this program and those who are chosen would use that opportunity to give back and apply what he learns to his students" (J. Bernard, personal communication, December 2, 2015). Both Fiorella and Bernard experienced life-changing opportunities through these sport diplomacy initiatives and are but two of hundreds of other youth, coaches, and sport administrators having similar experiences annually.

Envoy Program

In some ways, SportsUnited's Sports Envoys program is the opposite of the visitors program, as its goal is to accomplish improved cultural relations by sending athletes and coaches from the United States to foreign countries as ambassadors. Partnering with the U.S. Olympic Committee, U.S. sports federations and professional leagues, the envoy program identifies successful American athletes and former athletes who represent the country on foreign soil. Developed through U.S. embassies and consulates, delegates run sport camps and clinics, engaging with young athletes in important conversations surrounding the power of sport, leadership, and diversity. More than 150 athletes and teams have traveled to over 75 countries since the envoy program was established in 2007 ("Sports Envoys," n.d.).

A look inside. With a sparkling career that included an Olympic gold medal, World Cup title with the United States national soccer team, and two NCAA national championship titles as a North Carolina Tar Heel, Tiffany Roberts Sahaydak's soccer memories capture more than a few historic events. But at the top of her list of favorites, in a moment both special and humbling for Sahaydak, is when she was on hand to witness a mini World Cup soccer tournament held for teenage girls in Recife, Brazil.

While traveling as a SportsUnited envoy in 2014, Sahaydak's appearance marked the very first time most girls in this area were allowed to play organized soccer. The U.S. Embassy in Brazil assisted the SportsUnited program in recruiting girls from the favelas to play in their own tournament, complete with genuine referee crews and on designated soccer fields. Sahaydak recalled one girl in particular, who spoke to her about their shared interest in music. Sitting on the sidelines, speaking through a translator, they bonded over their mutual love of music, sport, and common thread of being a female footballer. The young woman broke down into tears, overwhelmed that an athlete with such a career would sit with her as a friend. Sahaydak realized in that moment that "no matter the language, or how far I was from home, here I was able to share two amazing things with this young woman: we both love futbal, and we are both girls."

Sahaydak recalls from another SportsUnited-sponsored trip the image of being in the middle of a field in the Philippines, with teammate Linda Hamilton, watching vehicles full of boys drive around the corner to participate in their session. Most players came shoeless or wearing their only pair. Often games were played barefoot to respect the reverence afforded to shoes, reserved solely for school. Here Sahaydak and Hamilton's presence marked the first time most boys had seen women play sports. While taking questions after the session, Sahaydak was struck by the boys' concern that her family viewed her as a disappointment for being a female athlete, and that many were surprised to find she was married. Sahaydak noted, "I felt a new responsibility to increase perspective through the vehicle of sports." Each trip allowed the chance to impart a positive message off the field, taking the empowering and diplomatic nature of soccer from the fields and into the minds of youth.

Playing for the US women's soccer team gave Sahaydak the chance to travel the world, playing in over 60 games in countries such as Sweden, Canada, and Portugal. But Sahaydak says emphatically, the SportsUnited trips have been life changing. Each time I come back even more grateful for the chance I had to bond with people around the world. It truly shows you the power of sport, so much so that a country can use it as an instrument for international relations (T. Roberts Sahaydak, personal communication, November 25, 2015).

Currently raising two daughters with husband Tim Sahaydak, associate head coach at the University of Central Florida, she has no interest in curbing her travel. "It's been a privilege to see the world, assist in empowering women and youth, and to teach my sport. The goal now is to make it an entire family affair" (T. Roberts Sahaydak, personal communication, November 25, 2015).

Grants Program

The Sports Grants program is the publicly available branch of the SportsUnited program, with opportunities open to any with interest in applying. Titled the International Sports Programming Initiative (ISPI), annual funding announcements call for proposals from public and private nonprofit organizations in the United States that address one of several sport-focused themes ("Sports Grants," n.d.). Covering topics such as sport for social change, sport and health, sport and disability, or sport and the environment, organizations may apply for these grants with an overarching goal of utilizing sport for diplomatic purposes (e.g., opening lines of communication, increasing mutual understanding). Each year the State Department identifies a list of countries, ones the U.S. government has high interest in building diplomatic relations, and with whom U.S. organizations can partner in developing these two-way exchanges.

A look inside. Humbly born out of a dining room in 1985, the National Ability Center (NAC) saw its vision coming to fruition when 18 of its athletes participated in the 2014 Paralympic Games in Sochi, Russia. Long departed are the early days as the Park City Handicapped Sports Association, subsisting on a $3,500 grant from the Disabled American Veterans of Utah to fund just 45 adaptive ski lessons. The National Ability Center, grown from the house of Meeche White and Peter Badewitz, capped the 2015 year, facilitating over 28,000 lessons for 4,800 individuals in sports such as horseback riding, snow sports, archery, water sports, and cycling. Located on a 26-acre campus in Park City, Utah, the NAC provides a spectrum of adaptive sports programs from beginner to competition and beyond. Its growth has focused on families as well as the military, through programs that develop and encourage independence, health, and wellness. Foreign growth in the adaptive sport field has also risen, supported in part through the NAC's work with various international organizations. Through two-way exchanges, American NAC mentors travel abroad, working hands-on with instructors in their home countries. Return exchanges bring instructors to the United States, often receiving their first exposure to true accessibility, in accessible walkways, doors, buildings, and vehicles. These opportunities exist in large part because of the U.S. Department of State's SportsUnited grants program.

Recently, Meeche White, now serving as an International Ambassador for NAC, traveled to Mexico to oversee a partnership between the NAC and DIF, Mexico's social service agency, to offer an adaptive horseback riding training program. This recent program brought equestrian instructors together for best practice training in adaptive sports. The session showed instructors how to nurture individuals from sitting passively, paired with a volunteer in the saddle, to riding independently with the assistance of side walkers. Meeche recollects, "The energy in the facility changed completely; riders were ecstatic, their parents were thrilled, and even the horses seemed more energetic with the empowering change in dynamic" (M. White, personal communication, November 30, 2015). Flipping the script on disabilities is something Meeche has seen the NAC do on a regular basis. She notes, "Once someone participates in physical activity, who has previously been told being in a wheelchair means only watching TV, they suddenly can see a future that also includes college, travel and sports. These are magical changes that occur" (M. White, personal communication, November 30, 2015).

The NAC is one example of an organization that is able to do more by working with SportsUnited through their grants program. In addition to supporting positive change in the disabled community, programs such as these allow for interactions between groups of people from the United States and other nations, having a powerful diplomatic impact as well. Groups of individuals who would never have the opportunity to interact with one another are brought together in working toward a common goal (in this case, sport and disability), and the impact on each individual is noticeable.

Global Sports Mentoring Program

The final and most recently established prong of SportsUnited programming is the Global Sports Mentoring Program. Recognizing the need for empowered girls and women, and the valuable role sport can play in accomplishing this, the Empowering Women and Girls Through Sports Initiative was officially launched in 2012 ("The Story Behind," 2014), which strongly utilized mentoring relationships as its base. The program has achieved huge success in building strong mentoring relationships between female senior executives in U.S. sport organizations and female sport leaders around the world. Annually, a cohort of approximately 15 foreign sport leaders are identified and hand-selected by U.S. Embassies to spend one month in a mentoring placement with a female executive in the United States. Leveraging a strategic partnership with ESPNW, SportsUnited is able to secure the highest level sport executives in the US as well as tell their story to a broader audience.

While in the U.S., mentees not only learn important lessons in business, education, media, and outreach, but are also aided in developing their own action plans, which are implemented upon return to their home countries. Women from over 40 countries have traveled to the United States and back home since the program's establishment in 2012. The application of the action plans has led to increased sport opportunities for girls and women in countries where they do not always exist. Some of the important results that have come through the Global Sports Mentoring Program include newly introduced legislation concerning rights for women and girls, opportunities for girls to play new sports or previously male-dominated sports, the establishment of values-based and leadership-based sport initiatives, activities for underserved populations (physical and mental disabilities, orphans), consideration of women's commissions within Olympic Committees, the development of girls-only tournaments and leagues, and a host of other education-based and after-school programming specifically aimed at empowering women and girls. Building on this success, the Global Sports Mentoring Program has grown to include a second mentoring program in 2016, focusing on sport and disabilities.

A look inside. Currently, Grace Chirumanzu is one of only four female sports reporters in Zimbabwe. She uses her blog and newspaper outlets to uplift female athletes, even when they have poor performances, saying, "It is not my job to destroy someone's personality, but to be constructively critical and to build them up" (U.S. Department of State, 2016). She personally believes it is the responsibility of media to highlight and inspire other women to take up sport, "I can be a voice for the voiceless" (U.S. Department of State, 2016). Following her experience at ESPN through the Global Sports Mentoring Program, she continues to work for equity in sports coverage for women and girls. "Women deserve to have their voices heard. I want to be the voice for the voiceless. I want to become the first female sports editor in Zimbabwe" (U.S. Department of State, 2016).

Tashi and Nungshi Malik were the first siblings and twins to complete the Adventurer's Grand Slam, which entails a summit of the seven highest peaks on each continent, and reaching the North and South Poles. The sisters were born in the state of Haryana in northern India, where their father bucked traditional gender norms, and signed his daughters up for a basic course in mountaineering. In India, women are valued for domestic skills, but are deemed incapable or unfit for athletics and physical activity. As Tashi said, "Women are born with mountains to climb, and that has become our inspiration for climbing the mountains outside" (U.S. Department of State, 2016). Accomplished activists, Tashi and Nungshi have spoken throughout India on women's empowerment, highlighted with a TEDx talk, and additionally have been honored by the President of India and the Chief Ministers of Uttara-khand, Haryana, and Delhi. Tashi and Nungshi hoped to utilize the Global Sports Mentoring Program to learn more about marketing, sports management, and fundraising. "Although we have ideas on how to approach our plans, we lack experience on a larger scale," Nungshi says. "We're novices in terms of entrepreneurship, and we know we'll have the opportunity to learn from women with an abundance of experience" (U.S. Department of State, 2016).

Born to a sports-minded family in Ankara, Turkey, Deniz Cengiz was drawn to rowing. Additionally, Deniz immersed herself in volunteer work, focusing heavily on tutoring orphans. This life pursuit eventually led her to be the Grassroots Program Development Officer for the Turkish Football Federation, advocating for disadvantaged youth and persons with disabilities. Deniz is responsible for arranging soccer tournaments and leagues for athletes who are deaf, blind, or have physical or mental disabilities, as well as juvenile prisoners, orphans, and at-risk youth. Her programs have served more than 60,000 people per year, at 60 different events across 45 Turkish provinces in the last five years alone. The

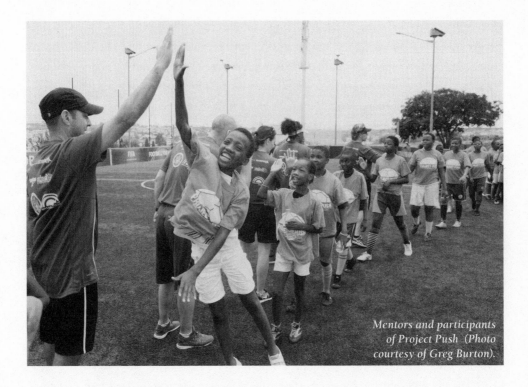

Mentors and participants of Project Push (Photo courtesy of Greg Burton).

Global Sports Mentoring Program played a large part in this, giving her expertise and networking in areas that would be critical to growing her programs in size and scope to reach even more disadvantaged youth.

WHY SPORT DIPLOMACY WORKS

The success of ping-pong diplomacy in paving the way for peaceful conversations between two previously warring countries brought to light the power of sport diplomacy. The U.S. government recognized the ability of sport to bring people of different nations together under peaceful circumstances, which could be a catalyst for change. One of the reasons sport worked in building Sino-U.S. relations in the 1970s was that sport was considered "neutral ground." Compared to direct politics or official government meetings, sport was considered a more low-risk testing ground for improving cultural relations (Goldberg, 2000; Murray, 2013; Walters, 2007). Through ping-pong diplomacy, sport became a new option for political advancement, one that the U.S. government need not overlook.

> If the playing field can provide a stage for political grievance and conflict, certainly it can also facilitate cooperation and understanding. Sports are now free from the tensions and limitations of the Cold War, allowing them to play a new, positive role in international politics. (Goldberg, 2000, p. 65)

The shift from purely political tactics to the more "soft" approach through sport seemed to come in response to other strategies' lack of success (Murray, 2013). Sport diplomacy, in many ways, happened unexpectedly through the positive path that ping-pong diplomacy was able to forge. It emerged partially as a result of "the recognition that the orthodox policies of 'development' have failed to deliver their objectives" (Levermore & Beacom, 2009, p. 1). At times when governments are on unsteady ground with one another or are testing the waters of improved relationships, sport can provide that opportunity. "Sport—and these sport-in-development initiatives—has been credited with being a very useful and non-political vehicle to bring disparate and often opposing groups in the development policy-making process together" (Levermore & Beacom, 2012, p. 2).

Sport itself is also continuing to increase in power, scope, and appeal (Murray, 2013), making it an ever-popular change agent. Because of the increased popularity of sport, sport and the media have an intricately intertwined relationship. In 2012, ESPN ranked as the world's most valuable media property at $40 billion (Badenhausen, 2012), and social media usage (e.g., Twitter, Facebook, Instagram, YouTube) among sport fans is off the charts. In 2013, 12 of the top 20 most-tweeted-about broadcasts during the year were sporting events (DiMoro, 2015). The media buy-in to sport makes it ever-appealing in terms of forging diplomatic relations. Sending Olympians and professional athletes to foreign countries on sport diplomacy efforts is all but guaranteed to garner media attention both in the United States and in the other country. Therefore, when the NBA, in collaboration with the U.S. Department of State, sends an envoy delegation of players and coaches to Myanmar, as they did in 2012, the media extensively covers the trip from sport, human interest, and political angles (Associated Press, 2012). The media's love for sport allows stories to reach more individuals than would be possible through other means. Reinforcing this, in March of 2016, President Obama traveled to Cuba for a diplomatic relations trip, which purposefully coincided with an exhibition baseball game between the Cuban National Team and MLB's Tampa Bay Rays (Oppmann, 2016).

Sport's inherent nature makes it an ideal diplomacy tool as well. Sport demonstrates that people of different nations are so very alike, while also uniquely different (Goldberg, 2000). Sport is symbolized by both competition and cooperation simultaneously. Therefore, it can be particularly useful in diplomacy efforts as "it can indicate that a country is strong and not to be trifled with, but that is it also flexible and amenable to negotiations" (Peppard & Riordan, 1993, p. 9). Additionally, the success of sport exchanges depends on the ability of administrators and coaches from different countries and cultures to work together effectively in making them happen. This important cooperation mirrors that which must exist for successful diplomatic relations, so is a fitting launching point to open the dialogue.

Finally, there is a uniqueness to the structure of sport in the United States that makes it an engaging diplomacy tool when interacting with other nations. Unlike most other nations, the US does not have a ministry of sport, does not support its Olympic athletes through government funding, and its professional leagues do not report to the U.S. government (Walters, 2007). The majority of other nations competing in the Olympic Games are organized through a ministry of sport, where funding of all athletes, coaches, and programs comes directly from the government. In the United States, the Olympic Committee is completely privately funded from sources such as broadcast rights, sponsorships, ticketing, licensing, and private donations ("Revenue Sources," 2015). This structure, while challenging at times, mirrors the capitalistic nature upon which the United States was founded. Therefore, the success of U.S. Olympians is a microcosm of what democracy and freedom allow society to achieve through hard work and determination (Walters, 2007). In this way, citizens of other nations who engage with the United States through sport learn about the values and characteristics that U.S. citizens embody. In the same vein, U.S. citizens are able to learn valuable lessons about foreign countries through their means of organizing and implementing sport.

As an example, in 2010-2011, the Center for Sport Leadership at Virginia Commonwealth University secured funding through SportsUnited's Sports Grants program to carry out a soccer coaching and life skills development initiative with the Shanghai Sports Bureau in Shanghai, China. Through this program, 12 coaches and administrators from the Shanghai Soccer Club spent two weeks in the U.S. working with coaches and professors on an intensive training program. Approximately one year later, six U.S. citizens who had worked with the Chinese coaches traveled to Shanghai to work with more coaches and youth on leadership and life skills development through soccer. In analyzing the program's impact, many themes emerged. However, chief among them was the strong impact that was made on both groups of delegates in terms of how these visits, and soccer itself, taught them so much about the other society in general.

For instance, the Chinese coaches reported having a significantly changed impression of American society by visiting for two weeks (LeCrom & Dwyer, 2013). Before the trip their impressions were based on American movies and the media; afterwards, they viewed America as a free society with limitless opportunities. Additionally, by working with and observing coaches working with their youth, the sport diplomats saw that coaching was reflective of each culture. Chinese visitors mentioned that American coaches work with their athletes in a much more flexible way, utilizing guided discovery as a tactic where the youth learn to make decisions on their own. One specifically commented, "I think what I learned here is the teaching methods, how you inspire the students. How we [Chinese coaches] teach is that they don't use their own [mind]; we just tell and they accept" (LeCrom & Dwyer, 2013, p. 9). This cultural difference, which manifested itself on the soccer field, was reflective of the open lines of communication between players and coaches in the United States (free speech). The more rigid, one-way form of communication that was observed between coaches and players in China mirrors their respect-based society, where adults are to be respected no matter what, so the system is much less participatory.

Clearly demonstrated through this example, sport is a powerful teaching tool, and one that can forge strong bonds and communicate subtle nuances of a culture or nation. While politics were not discussed during the exchange, both groups of delegates, as well as those they brought their experiences back to, learned much about citizens of the other country. Therefore, the goals of the program and of the U.S. Department of State (to increase cultural understanding between citizens of the United States and China) were clearly achieved. More than that, sport was successfully utilized as a teaching tool, providing support for sport diplomacy as a worthwhile and strategic endeavor in moving beyond one's own borders.

THE FUTURE OF SPORT DIPLOMACY IN THE UNITED STATES

In 2001, recognizing the potential sport has to be a successful engine for development and diplomacy, the United Nations (UN) created a position and designated the first-ever Special Advisor to the UN Secretary General on Sport for Development and Peace (Beutler, 2008). Two years later they commissioned a report titled "Sport for Development and Peace: Towards Achieving the Millennium Development Goals," recommending that sport be fully integrated and utilized as a development tool (Beutler, 2008; Kidd, 2008). The UN then designated 2005 the International Year of Sport and Physical Education. The timing of the UN's recognition of sport as a powerful development tool coincided directly with the United States' formal adoption of sport as an important diplomatic change agent.

The U.S. Department of State has added more programming and more funding over the past decade, demonstrating its belief in and commitment to sport as a powerful tool for diplomacy. While the U.S. Department of State is credited with leading this effort because they have a formalized sport-based program, it is not the only U.S. government agency engaging in this important work. The Pentagon and the Department of Defense have similar sport diplomacy initiatives in place related to peace-building and peace-keeping missions. The United States Agency for International Development (US AID) has awarded funding and programming to myriad sport-based initiatives. With an overall goal of "ending extreme poverty and promoting the development of resilient, democratic societies that are able to realize their potential," sport can be, and has been, a strong catalyst in these efforts ("Who we are," n.d.).

So what does the future hold in regard to the U.S. government's role in sport diplomacy? The short answer: a lot of potential. Historically, some of the very first delegations to visit nations that the US considered nations of concern were athletes (e.g., China, Cuba, Iran). These people-to-people exchanges with high media coverage tended to have more initial success than business-to-business or military-to-military interactions in opening up lines of communication. They were neutral testing grounds that allowed the US to make initial contact and assess next steps. They allowed the US to reach countries that they otherwise might not—sometimes because they are not yet willing to reach out in a directly political way.

Additionally, the focus of the SportsUnited program has been primarily on youth, ages 7-17, which is a strategic decision. If we are able to reach, teach, and engage with youth in a positive way, that information will have a multiplier effect when taken back to their families and communities. The youth are the future leaders of their countries—the ones who will be driving their nation's economy, making policy decisions, and influencing the next generation. Research shows that educating youth, especially girls, could lead to significant personal and societal benefits. If youth in low-income countries obtain basic reading skills, world poverty could be reduced by 12% (Gallucci, 2012). Additionally, low- and middle-income countries collectively lose approximately $92 billion per year due to uneducated girls (Gallucci, 2012). These statistics point to the importance of sport as both a diplomatic and developmental tool, which can be achieved simultaneously. The continued focus on youth in sport diplomacy initiatives bodes well for decades to come.

Still, sport diplomacy is not a magic bullet and is far from the only way to increase international relations. One criticism of sport diplomacy in general is its sustainability. Many sport-based diplomacy efforts are one-time visits or short-term exchanges between countries, with little long-term interaction or continued relationships. And while sustainability is often mentioned as a shortfall of sport-based efforts, very few address ways of working toward sustainable sport-based programming. LeCrom and Dwyer (2015) proposed a model for successfully coordinating sport diplomacy programs, noting three critical components: sustainability, integrated cultural experiences, and solid evaluation efforts. The authors stated, "this component [sustainability] must be developed from the beginning and it must be central in all decision-making, as it serves as the foundation for the lasting legacy of the program" (LeCrom & Dwyer, 2015, p. 661).

The SportsUnited program, while primarily composed of short-term programming, requires the embassies, grantees, visitors, and envoy diplomats to work sustainability into each and every program. For instance, in the grants program, grant review criteria state that "applicants must provide a plan to conduct activities after the Bureau-funded project has concluded in order to ensure that Bureau-supported programs are not isolated events" (U.S. Department of State, 2015). Essentially, the U.S. government-sponsored programs are one piece of the diplomatic puzzle, but cannot work alone. Schulenkorf (2010) advocates for similar collaborative efforts, calling sport diplomacy a starting point that must be integrated into larger social agendas for success to emerge.

In closing, sport has a bright future and secure place in the world of diplomacy. The U.S. government's continued commitment to sport diplomacy demonstrates the value seen in this powerful tool. Including athletes (and coaches and sports administrators) as diplomats allows the U.S. government to increase the size of its diplomatic core and to reach people through a beloved medium: sport. Goldberg summed it up well in stating,

> Sports are not a cure for animosities and conflicts that have existed for 50 years, but the success of the likes of Michael Jordan, Mark McGwire, Jesse Owens, or Pele can have positive effects beyond the playing field, onto the political chessboard. (2000, p. 69)

DISCUSSION QUESTIONS

1. What countries might the US think about in terms of engaging them through sport diplomacy? Why? What programs might work well in those countries, based upon what you know about their culture, sport interests, and political pursuits?

2. Beyond the U.S. Department of State, what are some other governmental agencies that might be able to successfully implement a sport diplomacy program? How might one go about doing this?

3. What might be some drawbacks to the U.S. government fully engaging in sport diplomacy? What would be some strategies for minimizing these drawbacks?

4. Based upon what you read about the four prongs of the Department of State's SportsUnited program, which do you think has the ability to find the most success? Why?

5. List some strategies to increasing the sustainability of SportsUnited-sponsored programs.

6. How do you see technological innovations changing how sport diplomacy programs can or may be implemented in the future?

7. SportsUnited focuses on people-to-people sport exchanges, where there is one-on-one interaction between people from the United States and other nations. How might one go about increasing the multiplier effect (spreading of lessons learned beyond those directly affected) that could come from these programs?

CLASS ACTIVITY/ASSIGNMENT

International Sports Programming Initiative

Based on the following information, put together a proposal for funding for a sport diplomacy initiative, funded through the U.S. Department of State's SportsUnited Grants Program. Identify a local in-country partner organization (in one of the foreign countries listed below) that will help facilitate the in-country aspects of the program. Your proposal must include the following:

1. Executive summary
2. Project narrative matched to the review criteria, including but not limited to
   a. Program description
   b. Program partners
   c. Participant selection criteria
   d. Evaluation plan
3. Inclusive timeline of activity (prior, during and after)
4. Comprehensive budget

Department of State: SportsUnited:
International Sports Programming Initiative (ISPI)

Eligible partner countries and territories in each region:

- Africa: Ethiopia, Mozambique, Nigeria, Rwanda, South Africa, Tanzania
- East Africa and the Pacific: Burma, Peoples Republic of China, Indonesia, Malaysia, Philippines
- Europe and Eurasia: Bosnia and Herzegovina, Cyprus, Georgia, Kosovo, Russia, Turkey

- Near East and North Africa: Algeria, Israel, Jordan, West Bank/Gaza
- South and Central Asia: India, Kazakhstan, Sri Lanka, Turkmenistan, Uzbekistan
- Western Hemisphere: Colombia, El Salvador, Guatemala, Haiti, Honduras, Nicaragua, Uruguay

Funding Opportunity Description

Purpose: ECA's Sports United programs' mission is to bring people from the United States together with people from across the globe using sport as the link that fosters understanding, mutual respect and a shared vision of what the world can be.

Eligible Themes

Sport for Social Change

Exchanges will focus on the role sport can play in promoting more stable and inclusive communities, and as an alterative to antisocial behavior. Project goals should include the importance of leadership, responsibility, teamwork, health living, and self-discipline to demonstrate how organized sports can encourage youth to stay in school, prevent substance abuse and violence, and mitigate extremist voices.

Sport and Health

Exchanges will focus on increasing awareness among young people of the importance of following a healthy lifestyle. Project goals should aim to prevent substance abuse, enhance physical fitness in order to prevent illness, and raise the overall quality of life through sports.

Sport and Disability

Exchange should promote sport, recreation, and fitness programs for persons with disabilities. Goals should include improving the quality of life for persons with disabilities by providing affordable, inclusive sports experiences that build self-esteem and confidence, enhancing active participation in community life and making a significant contribution to the physical and psychological health of people with disabilities. Additionally, projects should aim to raise awareness of nondisabled people about contributions that persons with disabilities make to society.

Sport and the Environment

Exchanges will focus on using sport as a means to promote the U.S. government's environmental priorities, spread awareness of greening activities, and reach out to a widespread audience around the world on the importance of the environment. Project goals should engage youth and youth influencers in the practices of environmental sustainability through programs addressing an assortment of topics.

Approximate Award Range

$130,000-$225,000

Audience

The intended audience is non-elite youth from underserved communities, their coaches and sports administrators, and nongovernmental organizations working in their communities.

Timeline

Projects may range in length from 1-3 years depending on the number of project components envisioned, the country/region targeted, and the extent of the evaluation plan proposed. Organizations are encouraged to plan enough time after project activities are completed to measure project outcomes.

Monitoring and Evaluation

Proposals must include a plan to monitor and evaluate the project's success, both as activities unfold and at the end of the program. The Bureau recommends that your proposal include a draft survey questionnaire or other technique plus a description of a methodology to use to link outcomes to original project objectives. Successful monitoring and evaluation depend heavily on setting clear goals and outcomes at the outset of a program. Your evaluation plan should include a description of your project's objectives, your anticipated project outcomes, and how and when you intend to measure these outcomes.

We encourage you to assess the following four levels of outcomes, as they relate to the program goals (listed here in increasing order of importance):

- Participant satisfaction with the program and exchange experience.

- Participant learning, such as increased knowledge, aptitude, skills, and changed understanding and attitude. Learning includes both substantive learning and mutual understanding.

- Participant behavior, create actions to apply knowledge in work or community; greater participation and responsibility in civic organizations; interpretation and explanation of experiences and new knowledge gained; continued contacts between participants, community members, and others.

- Institutional changes, such as increased collaboration and partnerships, policy reforms, new programming, and organizational improvements.

Budget

Allowable costs for the program include the following:

- Travel. International and domestic airfare, visas, transit costs, ground transportation costs.

- Per diem. ECA requests realistic costs that reflect the local economy and do not exceed federal per diem rates.

- Interpreters. One interpreter is typically needed for every four participants who require interpretation. Include per diem and transportation as well.

- Consultants. Consultants may be used to provide specialized expertise or to make presentations. Honoraria rates should not exceed $250 per day.

- Room rental. Rental of meeting space should exceed $250 per day.

- Materials. Proposals may contain costs to purchase, develop, and translate materials for participants.

- Equipment. Applicants may propose to use grant funds to purchase equipment such as computers and printers. Costs for furniture are not allowed.

- Administrative costs. May include salaries for grantee organization employees, fringe benefits, and other direct and indirect costs per detailed instruction. Proposals are considered more competitive if administrative costs do not exceed 25% of the total requested grant funds.

Review Criteria

- Program planning and ability to achieve objectives
- Cost effectiveness and cost sharing
- Support of diversity
- Post-grant activities
- Monitoring and evaluation

REFERENCES

Associated Press. (2012). U.S. sends envoys to Myanmar. *ESPN*. Retrieved from http://espn.go.com/nba/story/_/id/8304113/us-sends-hoop-players-coaches-myanmar

Badenhausen, K. (2012, November 9). Why ESPN is worth $40 billion as the world's most valuable media property. *Forbes*. Retrieved from http://www.forbes.com/sites/kurtbadenhausen/2012/11/09/why-espn-is-the-worlds-most-valuable-media-property-and-worth-40-billion/

Beutler, I. (2008). Sport serving development and peace: Achieving the goals of the United Nations through sport. *Sport in Society, 11,* 359-369.

Chehabi, H. E. (2001). Sport diplomacy between the United States and Iran. *Diplomacy & Statecraft, 12,* 89-106. doi:10.1080/09592290108406190

DeVoss, D. A. (2002, April). Ping-pong diplomacy. *Smithsonian Magazine*. Washington DC: Smithsonian Institution.

DiMoro, A. (2015, July 2). The growing impact of social media on today's sports culture. *Forbes*. Retrieved from http://www.forbes.com/sites/anthonydimoro/2015/07/02/the-growing-impact-of-social-media-on-todays-sports-culture/

Gallucci, R. (2012, June 4). The power of educating girls. *The World Post*. Retrieved from http://www.huffingtonpost.com/robert-gallucci/the-power-of-educating-gi_b_1562635.html

Gerin, R. (2007). Diplomacy gets a sporting chance. *Beijing Review,* 14-15.

Goldberg, J. (2000). Sporting diplomacy: Boosting the size of the diplomatic corps. *The Washington Quarterly, 23*(4), 63-70.

Hunt, T. M. (2006). American sport policy and the culture cold war: The Lyndon B. Johnson presidential years. *Journal of Sport History, 33,* 273-297.

Itoh, M. (2011). *The origin of ping-pong diplomacy*. New York, NY: Palgrave Macmillan.

Kidd, B. (2008). A new social movement: Sport for development and peace. *Sport in Society, 11,* 370-380.

LeCrom, C. W., & Dwyer, B. (2013). Plus-sport: The impact of a cross-cultural soccer coaching exchange. *Journal of Sport for Development, 1*(2), 1-15.

LeCrom, C. W., & Dwyer, B. (2015). From evaluator to insider: An academic's guide to managing sport for development programmes. *Sport in Society, 18,* 652-668. doi:10.1080/17430437.2014.982542

Levermore, R., & Beacom, A. (2009). *Sport and international development*. Hampshire, UK: Palgrave MacMillan.

Levermore, R., & Beacom, A. (2012). *Sport and international development*. Hampshire, UK: Palgrave MacMillan.

Murray, S. (2013). Moving beyond the ping-pong table: Sports diplomacy in the modern diplomatic environment. *Public Diplomacy Magazine, 9,* 11-16.

Nixon, R. M. (1969). Address by Richard M. Nixon. (1969). *Joint congressional commit-tee on inaugural ceremonies*. Retrieved from http://www.inaugural.senate.gov/about/past-inaugural-ceremonies/46th-inaugural-ceremonies.

Oppmann, P. (2016, March 22). Obama engages in baseball diplomacy in Cuba. *CNN Politics*. Retrieved from http://www.cnn.com/2016/03/22/politics/obama-cuba-baseball-diplomacy/

Orlins, S. (2012, March 02). The evolving role of sports diplomacy. *China-US Focus*. Retrieved from http://www.chinausfocus.com/foreign-policy/the-evolving-role-of-sports-diplomacy/

Peppard, V., & Riordan, J. (1993). *Playing politics: Soviet sport diplomacy to 1992*. Greenwich, CT: JAI Press.

Revenue Sources and Distribution. (2015). Official website of the Olympic movement. Retrieved from http://www.olympic.org/ioc-financing-revenue-sources-distribution?tab=sources

Sanders, B. (2011). Sport as public diplomacy. USC Center on Public Diplomacy. Retrieved from http://uscpublicdiplomacy.org/pdin_monitor_article/international_sport_as_public_diplomacy

Schulenkorf, N. (2010). Sport events and ethnic reconciliation: Attempting to create social change between Sinhalese, Tamil and Muslim Sportspeople in war-torn Sri Lanka. *International Review for the Sociology of Sport, 45*, 273-294.

Sports Envoys and Sports Visitors. (n.d.). Bureau of Educational and Cultural Affairs. [Website]. Retrieved from http://eca.state.gov/programs-initiatives/sports-diplomacy/sports-envoys-and-sports-visitors

Sports Grants. (n.d.). Bureau of Educational and Cultural Affairs. [Website]. Retrieved from http://eca.state.gov/programs-initiatives/sports-diplomacy/sports-grants

Story Behind the Program, The. (2014). Empowering women and girls through sports: An initia-tive of the U.S. Department of State. [Website]. Retrieved from http://globalsportswomen.org/global-sports-mentoring-program

U.S. Bureau of Educational and Cultural Affairs. (n.d.). About ECA. [Website]. Retrieved from http://eca.state.gov/about-bureau

U.S. Department of State, Bureau of Educational and Cultural Affairs (2015). *Request for grant proposals: International sports programming initiative*. [Website]. Retrieved from https://eca.state.gov/files/bureau/fy15_nofo_ispi_international_sports_programming_initiative.pdf

U.S. Department of State & University of Tennessee Center for Sport, Peace, and Society. (2016). *Emerging leader: Grace Chirumanzu*. [Website]. Retrieved from https://globalsportsmentoring.org/global-sports-mentor-program/emerging-leaders/grace-chirumanzu/

U.S. Department of State & University of Tennessee Center for Sport, Peace, and Society. (2016). *Emerging leader: Tashi and Nungshi Malik*. [Website]. Retrieved from https://globalsportsmentoring.org/global-sports-mentor-program/emerging-leaders/tashi-and-nungshi-malik/

Walters, C. (2007, August 3). Sports diplomacy is the new comeback kid. *USC Center on Public Diplomacy*. [Website]. Retrieved from http://uscpublicdiplomacy.org/blog/070803_sports_diplo-mancy_is_the_new_comeback_kid/#.V1OEqWdGNts.email

Who we are: Mission, vision and values. (n.d.). United States Agency for International Development. [Website]. Retrieved from https://www.usaid.gov/who-we-are/mission-vision-values

3

CULTURECONNECT AND THE U.S. DEPARTMENT OF STATE: A GATEWAY TO THE FUTURE OF SPORT DIPLOMACY

OMARI FAULKNER

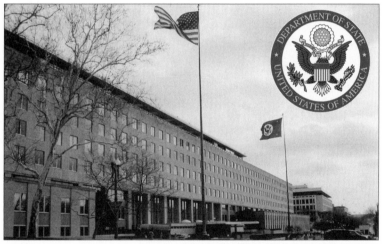

Photo courtesy: By Loren (Own work) [Public domain], via Wikimedia Commons.
US State Department Seal courtesy: U.S. Government [Public domain], via Wikimedia Commons

INTRODUCTION

On December 13, 2004, in the Treaty Room at the Department of State's Harry S. Truman Building, many foreign and State Department leaders highlighted the importance of cultural and sports diplomacy, cementing its impact as a foreign policy tool that would grow and prosper for generations to come. The event was an awards ceremony, honoring the international impact of the Department of State's Cultural Ambassadors and Sports Envoys. Secretary of State Colin L. Powell (2004b) was clear: "The epic stories of the American people are best expressed through the rhythms of our music and of our poetry, through the grace of our dancers and athletes."

Governments were once the single source of information for their citizens regarding foreign policy. They created the messaging and relayed the status of strategic relationships with international allies and adversaries. Today, the rise of social media and the growing importance of nonprofit organizations impose extraordinary demands on governments to respond to international events and changes in relationships. The new millennium brought swift innovations in how citizens receive information, creating in many cases more engaged global citizens. The strategic manner in which the U.S. Department of State united sports and diplomacy to communicate country values via cultural programs created a new pillar of diplomatic relations.

Soon after the terror attacks on September 11, 2001, the U.S. State Department created CultureConnect, an exchange program focused on building relationships through an elite group of leading American cultural figures to be known as Cultural Ambassadors (U.S. Department of State, 2004a). Investing in cultural and sports diplomacy proved that the United States saw international engagement as a priority. In May 2004, Secretary of State Colin Powell and Deputy Secretary of State Richard Armitage established the Cultural Envoys program, adding a new dimension to CultureConnect: an attempt to reach global youth through sports, utilizing previously unknown athletes.

CultureConnect's Envoy Program would utilize the talents of everyday Americans. Two recent graduates of Georgetown University, myself and my Georgetown University teammate Courtland Freeman, both basketball players, would embark on a mission to change how the United States engaged with the world's youth, particularly in the Arab world. It was the middle of a period where winning hearts and minds was a tall order, one that some State Department officials didn't think was best handled by recent college grads, but the Envoys program illustrated the importance of cultural diplomacy and of sports diplomacy to represent the very best of America, particularly its diversity.

THE CULTURAL AMBASSADORS PROGRAM

Governments around the world have traditionally communicated their nations' principles and cultural discriminators through the talents of globally respected artists, musicians, athletes, and more. Such figures quickly earn praise and mutual respect from others who also are comrades or aficionados of the art form or sport, and their ability to gain credibility and reach masses of people is often unmatched.

Patricia Harrison, Assistant Secretary of State for the Bureau of Educational and Cultural Affairs, created the CultureConnect program shortly after the terrorist attacks of September 11, 2001. In the face of grueling criticism, mostly as a result of America's invasion of Iraq, Assistant Secretary Harrison responded swiftly by assembling the Cultural Ambassadors Program, a group of professionals who exemplified the moral code of American freedom and diversity:

> a dedicated group of people known throughout the world for excellence in their
> fields who want to teach, mentor and work with young people. While overseas,
> they engage with youth by undertaking projects in their areas of expertise

through clinics, performances, coaching sessions, motivational speeches, master classes, and leadership training. (U.S. Department of State, 2004c)

The 2003-2004 cultural ambassadors were Debbie Allen (dance), Denyce Graves (opera), Michael Kaiser (arts leadership training), Dean Kamen (invention), Daniel Libeskind (architecture), Yo-Yo Ma (music), Wynton Marsalis (music), Frank McCourt (literature), Tracy McGrady (sports), Joel Meyerowitz (photography), Doris Roberts (television and film), Ron Silver (television and theater), and Mary Wilson (music).

The group covered all bases and cast a wide net, and all were well aware of the benefits of global interaction. Denyce Graves, one of the world's most accomplished opera singers, was already no stranger to international diplomacy when she agreed to a cultural ambassadorship, having been the only classical music artist invited to perform in a concert for the Nobel Peace Prize Awards show in Oslo, Norway. *USA Today* identified her as one of the "singers most likely to be an operatic superstar of the 21st century" (Graves, 2011). Yo-Yo Ma joined CultureConnect as an Ambassador in 2003. As one of the most famous cellists of all time, his passion for service had been recognized globally. During his travels most young musicians adored Yo-Yo Ma's diverse musical and cultural background. After moving to the US, one of his earliest public performances, at age 7, was for a gala event that included Presidents Eisenhower and Kennedy, and Leonard Bernstein (Huizeinga, 2015).

SPORTS DIPLOMACY

Sports have proven to connect people from all cultures and walks of life. From the 1950s through the 1970s, the U.S. government seized the opportunity to use athletics to enhance communication and dispel negative propaganda and stereotypes arising from the Cold War. In 1956, President Dwight Eisenhower, a former running back and linebacker for West Point, signed into law the International Cultural Exchange and Trade Fair Participation Act, expressing his vision that "little by little, mistrust based on falsehoods will give way to international understanding based on truth" (Library of Congress, n.d.). Between 1954 and 1963, more than 60 groups of athletes traveled to more than 100 countries to conduct clinics, play exhibition games, and engage with other nations. On December 25, 1957, Edward P. Eagan, then president and board chairman of the People to People Program, wrote, "Our athletes participating in international sport can help smooth the way for mutual understanding, peace on earth and good will to men" (Eagen, 1957, p.1).

The Department of State had not had a coordinated and funded sports diplomacy effort since the Cold War. In a 1983 *New York Times* sports editorial, Peter Ueberroth, then president of the Los Angeles Olympic Organizing Committee and later Commissioner of Baseball and the United States Olympic Committee chairman, addressed the lack of engagement through sports and called on the United States government to use sports diplomacy as public policy.

The United States government is sending $10,000 worth of basketballs, hoops and nets to the African nation of Burundi... The United States [instead] should

be sending coaches and athletes to Burundi and other countries to forge bonds of friendship and understanding throughout the world. (Uberroth, 1983)
He continued:

> The American people know that athletes influence our young people. We know, too, that it was competition between American and Chinese table tennis players a decade ago that opened the door for the establishment of diplomatic relations between the United States and China. But the United States government has not fully recognized sports as an ingredient of peace, as a chance to establish friendship and mutual understanding around the world....

> The United States cannot afford to continue to ignore the power of sports as a vehicle for world peace.... We urge the country's leaders to use athletes as emissaries of peace, friendship and understanding. Let's catch up with the rest of the world.

It was not covered as big news at the time, but it illustrates how far the United States had fallen behind other countries in making friends through sports.

The CultureConnect Ambassadors Program represented the beginnings of a revitalized sports diplomacy platform by engaging professional athletes who had worldly views and wanted to contribute diplomatically. Tracy McGrady, one of the National Basketball Association's most popular basketball players, was an original ambassador in 2004; the next year, New York Yankees center fielder Bernie Williams joined the elite group. He made a five-day trip to Colombia and Venezuela in which he squeezed in four baseball clinics; one concert (Williams is also a professional jazz guitarist); three exhausting workouts; dinner with Bill Brownfield, the United States ambassador to Venezuela; lunch with Colombian community leaders; an impromptu one-song performance; and autographs for thousands of people (Curry, 2005). His trip was extremely popular amongst the locals despite an ongoing tense political environment in both Colombia and Venezuela (Curry, 2005). Upon his arrival to Colombia, Mr. Williams was briefed by U.S. military, as Jack Curry (2005) reported: "The officer said there were 14,000 guerrillas who wanted to overthrow the government, 12,000 paramilitary soldiers who wanted to quell them, and uncertain number of Colombians who were ferocious about trampling anyone who interfered with their drug enterprises" (Curry, 2005)

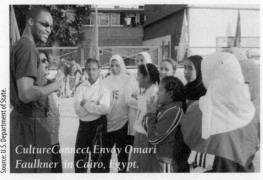

CultureConnect Envoy Omari Faulkner in Cairo, Egypt.

Source: U.S. Department of State.

Historically, American sports diplomacy efforts have centered on global games and well-known athletes. Secretary Powell also wanted to create more access and interaction with young athletes globally, so CultureConnect created the Cultural Envoy Program and picked my Georgetown University teammate Courtland Freeman and me to use "basketball to increase mutual understanding and illustrate some of the positive aspects of American culture, including teamwork, free expression and hard work" (U.S. Department of State, 2004b). As recent graduates of Georgetown, a campus nestled in Washington, D.C., with a strong tradition of foreign service, we both were fully aware, as were most students, of the international aftermath of the September 11 attacks. When given the opportunity to represent the United States and the game of basketball, we didn't hesitate.

A TENSE CLIMATE

In 2003, U.S. army soldiers and intelligence personnel committed human rights violations against detainees at the Abu Ghraib prison in Iraq. In 2004, vivid pictures and detailed reports of torture, rape, and humiliation dominated the media outlets and the international community was in an uproar. It was clear that U.S. soldiers committed heinous acts that United States government officials did not condone: Secretary Powell (2004a) said, "Our nation is now going through a period of deep disappointment, a period of deep pain over some of our soldiers not doing the right thing at a place called Abu Ghraib" (p.4). Americans were accused of waging war specifically against the Muslim faith. Nonstate organizations such as Al Qaeda amplified their efforts to target disenfranchised youth in the Muslim world, exploiting their lack of knowledge about America. Muslim nations all over the world were disgusted by the reports—disgust that terrorist organizations used to justify retaliation on the U.S. military and Americans overseas. As these organizations swelled and mobilized their efforts, the U.S. government began to increase their international diplomacy engagement, using culture as a tool for understanding.

Sports diplomacy was critical to U.S. diplomatic efforts in the wake of the release of the Abu Ghraib prison photos and subsequent investigation that understandably harmed our global image, especially in largely Muslim Bangladesh. Americans too were appalled and were determined to rebuild our image and prove that the prison scandal did not accurately reflect our democratic and human rights values (H. Thomas, U.S. Ambassador to Bangladesh, unpublished interview, November 15, 2015.).

The Risks Associated with Diplomacy

"You can't connect the dots looking forward; you can only connect them looking backwards. So you have to trust that the dots will somehow connect in your future," Steve Jobs said in a commencement addresss (Stanford Commencement Address, 2005, p.1).

The idea of two recent college graduates representing the U.S. government abroad presented risks on many fronts. Neither Freeman nor I were internationally renowned sports figures nor had we been confronted with anti-American audiences. But at the ages of 23 and 22 respectively, we represented a much-needed reprieve from the stereotypes that were being portrayed in the media. "What little exposure most participants had, if any, with Americans came in the form of U.S. diplomats wearing suits, who were generally further along in life, or whatever images they have seen on TV" (Freeman, 2015, p.2).

The State Department's approach was an original form of sports diplomacy, and the success of new programs cannot be determined until after execution of the program's goals, but within months, the significance of this innovative approach to sports diplomacy was apparent: Embassies across the globe were requesting the CultureConnect Envoy program, and the benefits (more participants) were immediately recognized. Events that were expected to be capped at 50 participants had to be adjusted on the fly to account for audiences ranging from 100 to 250. "My favorite experience was traveling with Omari and Courtland in Turkey," recalls Nicole Deaner, a public affairs specialist with the State Department.

> During that trip, we spent several days in Gaziantep, on the border of Syria. Our first stop was at a local stadium where we were expecting about 150 young people to show up for a basketball clinic. But much to our surprise, more than 700 young people showed up just to watch the basketball clinic and cheer for them. It was like being at a rock concert and Courtland and Omari were the rock stars—I couldn't believe it." (O. Faulkner, personal communication, November 22, 2015)

As envoys, we were reaching thousands at a time when understanding between young people was sorely needed—a period of war and division on multiple fronts.

"Only those who will risk going too far can possibly find out how far one can go."
—T.S. Eliot, *Preface to Harry Crosby, Transit of Venus, 1931*

WHY WAS THE ENGAGEMENT OF "AVERAGE AMERICANS" SO VITAL?

Accessibility and Relatability

In 2004, America needed to reengage the world in a conversation around its values and ideals. Sports diplomacy proved an effective method to build bridges of mutual understanding because sport is a global institution that connects people through nontraditional channels. The sporting arena comprises professionals, amateurs, and sporting aficionados. The latter group usually consists of fans, former players, and students of the game, and this is the group we primarily focused on during our travels.

The program aimed "to utilize the energy, skills and enthusiasm of talented, but lesser known Americans" to achieve its goals, and in this sense Freeman's and my youth made it a natural fit (U.S. Department of State, 2004b). We approached each trip with energy and enthusiasm for connecting with as many youth as possible, and the programming opportunities for the envoy program were limitless, unlike the ambassadors program, which had to take into account the demanding schedules of renowned artists and athletes. Within three months of the program's kickoff, the envoy program had worked in Bosnia, Romania, Albania, Turkey, El Salvador, Mexico, Brazil, Bolivia, Malaysia, Bangladesh, Sri Lanka, and India. Of even more significance, we visited multiple cities in each country, many of which had not had many U.S. visitors.

At an awards ceremony honoring the CultureConnect ambassadors and envoys, Secretary Powell graciously thanked the program for delivering results: "Reaching out to our world's youth is absolutely essential. They will inherit our world and be called upon to lead" (Powell, 2004b). In such a short period of time, it was evident to U.S. missions abroad that sports diplomacy had found its purpose. Subsequently, the United Nations began ramping up their Sports for Development portfolio, proclaiming 2005 as The International Year of Sport and Physical Education. The potential of sport to effectively convey messages and influence behavior on one hand, while improving the quality of people's lives and promoting peace on the other, has been increasingly recognized in recent years. As UN Secretary General Kofi Anan said, "Sport is a universal language that can bring people together, no matter what their origin, background, religious beliefs or economic status" (UN News Centre, 2004, p.1).

The impact of the program was immediately felt across the diplomatic community. Jamari Salleh, then a cultural affairs officer at the U.S. Embassy in Kuala Lumpur, said, "Courtland and Omari are opening doors for us with the future generations of Malaysia. This program needs to be continued if we are going to reap its long-term impact" (Deaner, 2004, p. 37).

A Two-Way Exchange

The Cultural Envoy Program was determined to engage youth in areas that had had little to no exposure to Americans and to welcome participants of all skill levels during basketball exchanges. This component was specifically important to the basic principles of cultural diplomacy programming. Cultural diplomacy is frequently described as "the exchange of ideas, information, art and other aspects of culture among nations and their peoples to foster mutual understanding" and this simplistic yet vital approach was a best practice for the Cultural Envoy Program (Cummings, 2009, p.1).

We approached each country and each program as an opportunity to learn as much as to teach. For example, while in Brazil, students performed traditional samba dances before one of our sports programs and taught us how to move to the rhythms. They all really enjoyed watching us samba, and we appreciated the cultural experience. On returning from the first Envoys tour through Eastern Europe, Courtland Freeman said,

> It's not just about basketball. We talk about music, about what college is like. We tell them to feel free to ask us questions about anything they want. They're dealing with a lot of the same issues we deal with: peer pressure and drugs and [the appeal of] criminal lifestyles. So we share our life experiences with them and tell them to listen to their parents and teachers and coaches and stay away from that route. (McIntosh, 2004, pg.1)

Basketball: A Global Game with American Roots

Although basketball is a thoroughly American game, it is becoming a world sport; there was a passion for basketball in every country we went to. "We also dealt with kids who don't play on a team but who love the game," Freeman said after returning from the 2004 tour through Albania, Bosnia, Romania, and Turkey (McIntosh, 2004, p. 1). Within nations where basketball ranked low on the list of most popular sports, the envoy program enticed the international sporting community because of the direct appeal to Western culture. The envoys traveled to some communities where basketball was unable to develop a strong appeal because of a lack of resources—due to poverty, declining sports facilities, or because locals lived and breathed soccer, cricket, and myriad other sporting activities.

In Brazil, camp participants placed the basketball on the floor and began joyfully kicking the ball up the court. Courtland and I saw this as an opportunity to learn more about soccer from the participants, so we paused our basketball drills to allow the young athletes to teach us. Spectators, media, and parents who had traveled more than 50 miles by multiple means of transportation just to learn more about the growing sport of basketball were thrilled to see U.S. Department of State representatives excited to learn soccer from locals.

Cultural Envoys in Dhaka, Bangladesh

The Envoy Program used basketball diplomacy as a tool to create a transparent environment that naturally encouraged groups to take risks, be open to different perspectives, and think outside the box. These groups included local government leaders, community activists, youth, and women, who in many countries were not afforded the equal opportunity to engage in sporting activities. The Cultural Envoy Program arrived in Dhaka, Bangladesh, in early October 2004, and one of the main focus areas was on encouraging the active participation of young girls, to increase their interest and to promote the continuation of the lifelong benefits of sports.

Although some claimed that young women in Bangladesh should focus on more pressing issues, the responses to Envoys working with young girls were excitement and welcome. Basketball was new to many Bangladeshis, as was having American visitors. During the visit, Harry Thomas (2015), the U.S. Ambassador to Bangladesh, made a profound observation as to the impact of the CultureConnect Program:

> Courtland and Omari's participation in sports diplomacy had an immediate and long-lasting impact on bilateral relations between Bangladesh and the United States. Few American athletes or entertainers venture to Bangladesh, an impoverished but democratic country of over 150 million people, many of whom are struggling to survive. In fact, during my tenure as U.S. Ambassador to Bangladesh (2003-2005), Omari Faulkner, Courtland Freeman and Mary Wilson, formerly of the Supremes, were the only Western athletes/entertainers who traveled to Bangladesh—others who visited [played] cricket and soccer, which are beloved games in the region. Little was known of basketball prior to Courtland and Omari's trip, but they were quickly able to engage the public with their kindness, easygoing manner and ability to capture the imagination of a broad spectrum of the public who initially gawked at their height. In teaching children a new game and convincing them that they could play it, Courtland and Omari helped young people gain

confidence. The important engagement they made was with young girls: In a country where cultural and religious habits often frown on women participating in sports, Courtland and Omari were able to teach girls to play. The U.S. Embassy worked with school headmasters and parents to promote girls' participation and helped to design culturally acceptable sports attire. Courtland and Omari's tutelage of girls was broadcast nationwide on TV and through social media, became a source of pride for the participants, and led to a much-needed national debate about sports participation for girls and women that continued long after their departure. (Thomas, 2015)

Months before the Envoy Program arrived in Dhaka, a flood covered more than 60% of the nation. Later, just weeks before the envoy arrived, 24 people were killed and more than 300 injured at an antiterrorism rally on August 21, 2004. This horrific event epitomized the volatile political environment in Dhaka. Such attacks have become commonplace in Bangladesh (Jamwal, 2004). Most claim it was a planned assassination attempt on Sheikh Hasina Wajed, the political leader of the Awami League, one of the largest political parties in Bangladesh.

Cultural climates such as those in Bangladesh were the exact focus of the Sports Envoy program, and the exchange of experiences and ideas was well received by both parties. It was an honor, for example, for Freeman and I to work with a group of eager young girls at Dhanmondi Wooden Floor Gymnasium. In such a setting, we had the opportunity to share stories beyond basketball and connect on a level that will someday help continue the growth of youth sports in Bangladesh, especially for women. These young women were very energetic, intelligent and optimistic about their futures—qualities that speak volumes about the bright future of Bangladesh, in sports as well as other arenas.

THE 2004-2005 CULTURAL ENVOYS, IN THEIR OWN WORDS:

Q: *What impact did your participation in the CultureConnect Envoy Program have on the participants?*

A: Working as a CultureConnect Sports Envoy allowed me to play an important role in the Department of State's mission to improve our image abroad. Discussing the valuable characteristics that basketball in particular and sports in general offer (i.e., teamwork, leadership, discipline, work ethic and time management), we held intimate conversations about life and the challenges young people face on a daily basis. I was candid about my own life, and what it was like for young people growing up in the US, and encouraged the participants to freely ask questions and discuss some of the challenges they faced. These discussions fostered an atmosphere of trust and understanding.

I used personal stories from my own life, and those of my friends, growing up in the US, to illustrate that Americans had to work very hard and make the right life choices in order to be successful, get an education, and become gainfully employed. I explained that while the U.S.

Continued

THE 2004-2005 CULTURAL ENVOYS, IN THEIR OWN WORDS:

Continued from page 47

is a prosperous country with great opportunities, people still had to work hard and struggle to reach their goals and utilize the opportunities it had to offer. Many young participants were surprised to hear that there was poverty, homelessness, and hunger in the U.S.

Another prominent stereotype that the program helped to dispel was the notion that the US was a monolithic country. Being an African American, I was asked by participants on more than one occasion if I were really American or if I were actually from Cuba or an African country. Many of our participants were from places where there was not any interaction with Americans, and the only thing they knew about the US were the images they saw in movies and the rumors they heard in their communities. I used those opportunities to highlight how diverse the US is and discuss our history and how far we have come as a nation since our independence over 200 years ago. Many participants were shocked to hear that the U.S. was made up of Americans of all religious and ethnic backgrounds who were able to coexist peacefully and work together to pursue a better country.

Having the freedom and latitude to talk about the rich cultural inclusion that takes place in the US while noting that it was not a Utopian society, and that discrimination and hatred still existed, went a long way in building trust with the participants. Many of the participants were unaware of U.S. history and the obstacles the nation has overcome in regards to equality and civil rights for all of our citizens. They were eager to hear about the progress the US has made and the examples of cooperation and togetherness across cultural, ethnic, and religious divides that exist throughout the US. They became hopeful that their own countries could see a future where its citizens work to overcome historical tensions and promote a sense of togetherness despite whatever differences may exist. We stressed that it was important for the participants to be leaders in their own communities and set a positive example for their younger relatives in order to help their communities and countries achieve the change they wanted to see (O. Faulkner, personal communication, December 10, 2015).

Q: *Describe your most memorable CultureConnect experience.*

A: My most memorable experience came in early July of 2004, when my feet touched the ground of another country other than the United States for the first time in my life. We arrived in Sarajevo, Bosnia, and Herzegovina to work directly with youth, sport coaches, and future community leaders. Not fully aware of how our program would be received, I was overwhelmed with nervousness and anticipation from the start. That would all rapidly change and I would see firsthand the power of sports.

Not far removed from civil war and ongoing internal conflicts, Bosnia and Herzegovina's rich cultural heritage overpowered the destruction that remained, and prevailed through unhealed hearts of war and division. We hosted one of our last basketball exchange programs in Brcko, a small town in the north of Bosnia. The community was divided into three ethnic groups that rarely collaborated peacefully: Bosniaks (Muslims), Croats (Roman Catholics) and Serbs (Orthodox Christians). From the very beginning of the program, the tension in the gym was palpable, and the youth participants were very apprehensive about working together during drills. They all clustered by ethnic group and did not venture from their pack.

Once this was confirmed by our language interpreter, we decided it would be advantageous to mix the teams by location and ethnic groups. This was not a popular decision at first; many of the parents and spectators seemed confused at the start. Courtland and I briefly explained our program goals, which consisted of three basic ground rules—work together, learn something new, and have fun. Within minutes, they were high-fiving their new teammates, cheering from the sidelines, and providing encouragement for the entire gymnasium, thus proving that the future of Bosnia and Herzegovina rested in the hands of youth who could, indeed, work together.

That moment will always stand out as one of my favorite moments of the CultureConnect program, because from the very beginning of our travels, it was apparent that we could have a significant impact. A woman who had traveled from a neighboring community to watch her granddaughter play basketball mentioned to me that she had a new view of America and a new view of the future of Bosnia. After she thanked me for coming to their town, I told her that it was a learning experience that would travel with me forever. That remains true today.

CONCLUSION

Under Secretary Powell's leadership, American sports diplomacy was reintroduced to the global community. In 2003, under Secretary Powell's leadership, support for sports diplomacy emerged from the top floor of the State Department in Washington, D.C., to U.S. embassies and consulates all over the world. This top-down approach had allowed for positive growth in the practical usage and the primary responsibility of implementation of sport as a diplomacy tool for engagement. After Secretary Powell retired, each of his successors has supported sports exchanges as a foreign policy framework for building relationships.

Further detailed in Chapter 2, the Educational and Cultural Affairs (ECA) bureau has a dedicated division solely responsible for sports diplomacy, called SportsUnited, tapping into the ability of sports to increase dialogue and cultural understanding between people around the world. Sports is a means to reach audiences with little to no exposure to American culture, providing a real life glimpse of America while highlighting our common values. Since the inception of the CultureConnect program, the State Department has also increased funding to address issues, such as equal rights for women and girls and economic development. Sport has been the catalyst for it all. By embracing the importance of sports diplomacy exchanges during times of peace, the US has invested in continuous outreach as a form of conflict prevention as well as engagement through its best asset—American people and culture.

DISCUSSION QUESTIONS

1. What was the purpose of the CultureConnect program?
2. Name advantages and disadvantages to engaging known and unknown athletes and representatives in sport diplomacy initiatives?
3. How can geopolitical and social tensions contribute to the success or failure of sport diplomacy initiatives between average citizens of two different nations?
4. Can top-down support affect the influence, reach, and sustainability of sport diplomacy initiatives? If so, how?

5. What were some of the effects on program participants, based on the examples provided throughout the chapter?

6. How could sport have reignited tensions during the programs that were held? What should be done in such a situation?

REFERENCES

Cummings, M. (2009, June 26). *Cultural diplomacy and the United States government: A survey.* Retrieved from http://www.americansforthearts.org/by-program/reports-and-data/legislation-policy/naappd/cultural-diplomacy-and-the-united-states-government-a-survey

Curry, J. (2005, February 18). Baseball: Plucking at a star's heartstrings. *The New York Times.* Retrieved from, http://www.nytimes.com/2005/02/18/sports/washington/baseball-plucking-at-a-stars-heartstrings.html?_r=0

Deaner, N. (2004, December). *Dribble, dunk and dialogue.* Retrieved from http://www.state.gov/documents/organization/191568.pdf

Eagan, E. P. (1957, December 25). *People-to-people sports committee incorporated.* Retrieved from http://www.eisenhower.archives.gov/research/online_documents/people_to_people/BinderB.pdf

Graves, D. (2011). *Critical Acclaim.* Retrieved http://www.denycegraves.com/criticalacclaim.aspx

Huizenga, T. (2015, October 7). *The diverse world of Yo-Yo Ma.* Retrieved from http://www.npr.org/sections/deceptivecadence/2015/10/07/446364616/the-diverse-world-of-yo-yo-ma

Jamwal, N. (2004, Jan-Mar). Border management: Dilemma of guarding the India-Bangladesh border. *Institute for Defence Studies and Analyses, 28,* 5-36. Retrieved from http://www.idsa.in/system/files/strategicanalysis_Jamwal_0304.pdf

Jobs, Steve (2005, June 12). *Stanford Commencement Speech.* Retrieved from http://news.stanford.edu/2005/06/14/jobs-061505/

Library of Congress. (n.d.). *Hope for America: Performers, politics and pop culture.* Retrieved from http://www.loc.gov/exhibits/hope-for-america/cultural-diplomacy.html

McIntosh, P. (2004, August 27). *Former U.S. college basketball stars initiate "Cultural Envoy" program.* Retrieved from http://iipdigital.usembassy.gov/st/english/article/2004/08/20040827174509eaifas0.2240259.html#axzz3uuw8z75n

Powell, C. L. (2004a). "Commencement address" Transcript from Wake Forest University, May 17, 2004. Retrieved from http://www.wfu.edu/wfunews/2004/051704transcript.html

Powell, C. L. (2004b). "Remarks at an awards ceremony honoring CultureConnect ambassadors and basketball envoys." Transcript of speech given at U.S. Department of State Convocation, December 13, 2004. Retrieved from http://2001-2009.state.gov/secretary/former/powell/remarks/39721.htm

Ueberroth, P. V. (1983, May 1). A call for the U.S. to catch up in sports diplomacy. *The New York Times.* Retrieved from http://www.nytimes.com/1983/05/01/sports/a-call-for-the-us-to-catch-up-in-sports-diplomacy.html

U.S. Department of State. (2004a, January 31). "About." [website]. Retrieved from https://web.archive.org/web/20040131052213/http://cultureconnect.state.gov/index.v3page?p=about

U.S. Department of State. (2004b, October 31). "CultureConnect—Cultural envoys program." [website]. Retrieved from https://web.archive.org/web/20041031134037/http://exchanges.state.gov/education/citizens/culture/envoys.htm

U.S. Department of State. (2004c, January 31). *Message from Patricia S. Harrison, Assistant Secretary of State, Bureau of Educational and Cultural Affairs.* Retrieved from https://web.archive.org/web/20040131052213/http://cultureconnect.state.gov/index.v3page?p=about

UN News Centre. (2004, November 4). "UN launches International Year of Sport and Physical Education." Retrieved from http://www.un.org/apps/news/story.asp?NewsID=12458&Cr=sport&Cr1#.VniSTJMrKHp

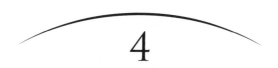

4

THE BELIZEAN YOUTH SPORT COALITION

PAUL WRIGHT · JENN JACOBS · JIM RESSLER · STEVEN HOWELL

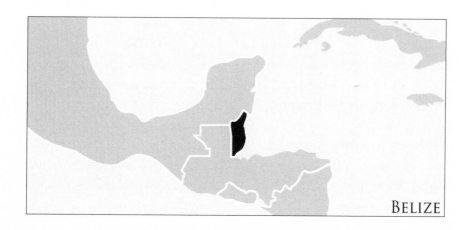

BELIZE

Sports have the power to change the world. It has the power to inspire, the power to unite people in a way that little else does. It speaks to youth in a language they understand. Sports can create hope, where there was once only despair. It is more powerful than governments in breaking down racial barriers. It laughs in the face of all types of discrimination.
—Nelson Mandela, *Laureus Sport Awards (2000)*

In this chapter, we describe the Belizean Youth Sport Coalition (BYSC) as a novel approach to sport for diplomacy. The BYSC has been funded by the United States Department of State Bureau of Cultural and Education Affairs through the SportsUnited: International Sports Programming Initiative, which enables nonprofit organizations to create programs where sport plays a role in promoting more stable and inclusive communities. As a result of this funding, we have supported the formation of a coalition of governmental and nongovernmental youth-serving organizations in Belize since 2013. We have trained administrators, coaches, teachers, and youth workers in coordination with the U.S. Department of State and the U.S. Embassy at Belmopan. The focus of this two-way exchange and training grant is promoting positive youth development and social change through sport.

While the BYSC fits within a sport-for-diplomacy agenda, it is unique in that it leverages the power of youth sport and integrates theory and practice from other fields, such as sport-based youth development and collective impact. In this chapter, we describe the Belizean context and ways the BYSC project aligns with U.S. national interests. We explain how the BYSC was designed to address specific contextual challenges and opportunities. Finally, we outline accomplishments to date and lessons learned that may inform other sport-for-diplomacy efforts.

SPORT FOR DIPLOMACY

In 2003, the United Nations passed Resolution 58/5, which officially recognized sport as an instrument for achieving peace, health, education, and economic development objectives. Sport has also been recognized as a vehicle for strengthening social and political relations between nations. Many international agencies support the use of sport for diplomacy, including the United Nations Sport for Development and Peace (2015) and the International Platform on Sport and Development (2015). These organizations emphasize the impact sport can have on bringing people together from different cultural and linguistic backgrounds to achieve social change. Sport for diplomacy is a timely and relevant topic because of its potential to promote peace and tolerance between people and nations.

The most well-known instance of sport being used for diplomatic efforts is the Olympics. The history of these games has showcased sport on an international stage with underlying principles of inclusivity, citizenship, cultural understanding, fairness, and teamwork (Jackson, 2013). The Olympics highlight the most traditional use of sport for diplomatic efforts, which includes fostering discussion and interaction between nations. This form of sport diplomacy brings people together for sporting events and presents opportunities to calm tensions or send a diplomatic message. Sport for diplomacy can also involve diplomatic efforts that lead to a sport competition between nations, or the negotiations and communication that allow sport exchanges to take place in a safe environment (Murray & Pigman, 2014). Using sport this way is more challenging to coordinate, and gaps in the literature reflect this challenge.

Despite significant research examining the influence of sport on politics and foreign policy, sport as a tool for diplomacy is less researched (Murray & Pigman, 2014). Most research on this topic includes specific cases between the US and nations such as Japan (Manzenreiter, 2008) and Iran (Chehabi, 2001). Manzenreiter (2008) explored how football (soccer) has been used as an international tool to advance intercultural relationships and define power relations and norms between countries. In Chehabi's (2001) study, sport was viewed as a tool to decrease tensions between Iran and the US; however, there were no observed lasting effects on the positive outcomes. Beyond these two seminal case studies, few attempts have been made to clarify the relationship between sport and diplomacy (Pigman & Rofe, 2014).

The appeal of sport as a remedy for conflict between nations derives from its nature for promoting play and friendly competition (Baker, Esherick, & Baker, 2011). Early research suggested close proximity and physical contact of players during team sporting events promote understanding and a lack of fear and discomfort (Allport, 1954). Through such interaction, sport may contribute to the development of collective identities where hostility is decreased and tolerance is fostered between societies. Sport is also seen as instrumental in enhancing health and well-being for people through supporting skill acquisition, identity development, and opportunities for self-efficacy (Lawson, 2005). Finally, sport is seen as a mechanism for advancing economies through its billion-dollar industry across the United States and other established nations (Pitts & Stotlar, 2007).

While significant research supports the influence that sport can have on lessening conflict and contributing to peace, it is argued sport can have a negative impact by fueling struggle and disagreement (Jackson, 2013). Sport programs lacking in design and implementation risk promoting negative outcomes such as violence, corruption, fraud, and a win-at-all-costs mentality (Lawson, 2005). Other programs fail to address social benefits beyond mere sport participation or to plan for sustainability (Spaaij, 2012). Some researchers argue the positive effects of sport are not automatic, but result from personal and social development in intentional ways (Crabbe, 2006; Hartmann & Kwauk, 2011; Petitpas, Cornelius, Van Raalte, & Jones, 2005).

One way to maximize the power of sport for diplomacy is to deliver programs that align with national and local campaigns so consistent themes are communicated. It is also recommended that sport-for-diplomacy initiatives focus on empowering people through a variety of program factors. For example, programs with a central focus for building local capacity are essential for fostering sustainability and long-term partnerships. Furthermore, research supports the idea of designing and delivering sport-for-diplomacy programs in conjunction with local input (Spaaij & Jeanes, 2013). Programs that rely too heavily on the expertise and perspective of the Global North often have issues related to power, transparency, and accountability because they overlook the importance of understanding the local context (Kidd, 2008). Instead, to advance developmental goals and sustain diplomatic effects, efforts should be coordinated to engage and empower participants and communities in a collaborative way.

SPORTSUNITED PROGRAM

Funding for the project described in this chapter came from SportsUnited, a program of the Bureau of Educational and Cultural Affairs (ECA) division of the U.S. Department of State. The history, structure, and mission of SportsUnited are explained in detail earlier in this book: see "The U.S. Government's Role in Sport Diplomacy" and "CultureConnect and the U.S. Department of State: A Gateway to the Future of Sport Diplomacy." Murray and Pigman (2014), describe SportsUnited as a strong example of the intentional and systematic use of sport for diplomacy, stating, "The U.S. Department of State, for example, typifies a rallying call 'to aggressively use sports as a diplomatic tool' through programmes like their SportsUnited initiative" (p. 1102). A recent study of SportsUnited programs (Bureau of Educational and Cultural Affairs, 2013) reported findings such as increased favorability toward and knowledge of the US, as well as knowledge gains in terms of democratic values in the US. Upon completion of programs, 80% of respondents or more reported "moderate" or "extensive" knowledge of freedom of speech, ethnic diversity, and religious diversity. In addition, coaches and program administrators have used skills they learned in the program to start new projects in their communities to address social problems and to promote inclusion of underserved populations. Roughly one-half (51%) of the foreign coaches and sports administrators surveyed reported that, after returning home, they were in contact with coaches they had met in the US, and many of those surveyed (87%) reported sharing their experience with others in their home countries.

BELIZEAN CONTEXT

Formerly British Honduras, Belize became an independent nation in 1984. According to the 2010 Census, Belize has a population of 312,698. The country's largest city and its capital, Belize City has a population just over 70,000. Although a small and fairly young nation, Belize has a rich history and vibrant culture. The majority of the population describes their ethnic background as Creole, Mayan, German, East Indian, or mixed; however, English is the official language. The economy is based primarily on tourism, which highlights coral reefs, archeological sites, and diverse flora and fauna. Major agricultural exports include sugarcane, citrus fruit, and bananas.

Challenges

Central America is a diplomatic priority region for the U.S. government. According to the Central America Regional Security Initiative (CARSI), this region has among the world's highest per capita murder rates as a result of rampant gang violence and organized crime rooted in the narcotics trade. Therefore, CARSI outlines goals related to social stability, good citizenship, and safer streets. Belize has been identified as a significant drug transit point along the Mexican border. Issues such as gang- and drug-related violence, poverty, and low educational outcomes common in Central America are evident in Belize. In fact, Belize's per capita homicide rate of 46 homicides per 100,000 inhabitants in 2012 ranks among the highest in the world (U.S. Overseas Security Advisory Council, 2013). At the beginning of Fiscal Year 2015, U.S. President Barack Obama released his annual presidential determination to Congress of major drug-transit and illicit drug-producing countries, which included Belize along with 21 other countries (Ramos, 2014). Clearly, the challenges facing Belize are serious and affect U.S. interests. For these reasons, the country was identified for targeted support through the SportsUnited program.

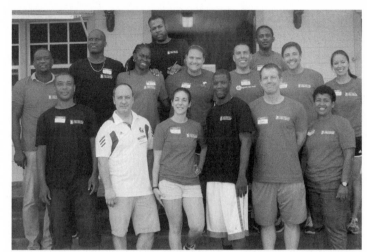

Members of the Belizean Youth Sport Coalition (BYSC) leadership team, including coach-trainers from Belize and professors and practitioners from Northern Illinois University.

Sport Culture

Sport has always been popular in Belize; however, due to gaps in financing, facilities, infrastructure, and training, the country has never been a major player at the international level. Belize participates in select events in the Olympics, the Commonwealth Games, and the Pan-American Games, but has won only two medals in these major international competitions: bronze in 1979 and 1983 for women's softball in the Pan American Games (Breaking News Belize, 2015a). The country also sends athletes to compete in the Special Olympics World Games and has medaled in bocce ball (Breaking News Belize, 2015b). Popular sports in Belize include basketball, soccer, cycling, track and field, and softball with these and other sports sanctioned and overseen by the National Sport Council (Ministry of Education, Youth, Sports, and Culture, 2015) which is under the government's Ministry of Education. There are no professional sport organizations in Belize, but basketball and soccer have semi-professional leagues.

Despite limited resources, sports continue to be an overarching and community-centralized theme in Belizean culture. For example, the annual La Ruta Maya Belize Endurance Canoe race is the longest race of its kind in Central America and is composed of 170 miles of paddling on the Belize River over the course of four days. Approximately 100 teams from countries such as Belize, Canada, Japan, United States, and United Kingdom participate annually. This event, which coincides with a Belizean federal holiday, attracts thousands of Belizeans and tourists annually, and includes live entertainment, food, games, and close-up views as the canoes pass. Cycling is another example of a longstanding sporting tradition. The Holy Saturday Cross Country Cycling Classic has been held on Easter weekend annually since 1928. Belizeans also take great pride in their individual athletes, who have excelled and achieved prominence in the region on the international stage, such as track-and-field star Marion Jones.

The government in Belize has struggled with major initiatives related to sport. For example, the previous Minister of Sport has been lambasted in the media for the government's inability to complete the Marion Jones stadium project, which began in 2009. After seven years, over $20 million spent, and several delays, the stadium is still incomplete (Channel 5 Belize, 2015a). As an example of diplomacy related to sport, the Mexican government has pledged to assist Belize by fully funding a multipurpose sports building that will be part of the Marion Jones Complex (Channel 5 Belize, 2015b). Belize also struggles to form a national sport policy. A call was released in 2012 for an external consultant to facilitate the formation of this policy. Work began in 2013 with limited input from sport organizations or the general public (Seven News Belize, 2013). At the time of this writing, a national sport policy has yet to be produced.

Youth in Belize

Belize has a young population, with over 56% of the country's citizens under 24 years old (United States Central Intelligence Agency, 2015). This demographic profile, coupled with high levels of school drop-out and low educational outcomes, presents a need for alternative activities to increase education and leadership opportunities for youth. To be effective, such activities must be appealing to youth and promote social development, self-confidence, leadership, and civic participation. Research shows intentionally designed programs can promote qualities that enable youth to succeed in school and contribute to their community in positive ways (Durlak Weissberg, Dymnicki, Taylor, & Schellinger, 2011; Peterson, 2013). Related to these needs and opportunities, Belize has established a National Youth Development Policy (Youth Policy, 2013), which centers on three goals: (a) empower and support young people in achieving optimal well-being in a supportive environment; (b) ensure comprehensive policies and institutional frameworks are multisectoral, coordinated, cohesive and resourced; and (c) create an "optimal ecology" of home, school, and community that provides young people a positive climate to grow up healthy, caring, and responsible. Despite the potential for sport to contribute to these youth development goals, youth sport in Belize is lacking in facilities, resources, and structure. In fact, many Belizeans insist that the nation's limited success competing at the international level stems from the lack of a coordinated approach to providing high quality youth sport programming.

BELIZEAN YOUTH SPORT COALITION

The BYSC project was proposed to address the U.S. diplomatic objectives in a way that aligned with the needs, opportunities, and pressures seen in Belize. Our program has been developed in conversation with multiple youth-serving agencies in Belize, including the YMCA of Belize, the National Sport Council, the Ministry of Education, Youth and Sports, and the Belize City Council. We also sought input from the SportsUnited program officer, an In-Country Coordinator (ICC), and the Public Affairs Section at the U.S. Embassy in Belmopan. Based on initial feedback and continuous refinement, our approach has been tailored to the local context (Kidd, 2008; Spaaij & Jeanes, 2013) As a sport-for-diplomacy project, the BYSC is unique because of its focus on youth development, intentional training, and capacity building for collective impact. To improve the program and address gaps in the literature, we have also invested significant time and effort in evaluation (Murray & Pigman, 2014). The rationale for these decisions and their influence on the project are described in the following sections.

Positive Youth Development

As explained above, more than one-half of the population in Belize is under the age of 18. This segment of the population is most likely to become involved in narcotrafficking, gang involvement, criminal activity, and the other social problems facing Belize (U.S. Overseas Security Advisory Council, 2013; Ramos, 2014). It stands to reason any initiative to spark social change in Belize should focus on the youth population. This logic is reflected in CARSI initiatives and the priorities of the U.S. Embassy at Belmopan that call for positive alternative activities for youth in Belize. However, research shows youth programs that focus only on deficit reduction are not as effective as those that take a more holistic, positive, and developmental approach (Catalano et al., 2004; Hellison & Cutforth, 1997). In fact, a meta-analysis of findings from over 60 studies (Durlak, et al., 2010) demonstrated that high quality, extracurricular youth programs designed to promote personal and social skills in children and adolescents contribute to improved grades in reading and math, improved school attendance, reduction in problem behaviors, improved academic achievement, increased positive social behavior, and more positive school engagement.

Youth development scholars contend benefits such as those listed above can be attributed largely to social and emotional learning and the development of transferable life skills (Greenberg et al., 2003; Newman & Dusenbury, 2015). For example, youth who learn the value of persistence and effort are more likely to have improved attendance and homework completion in school. Those who learn to control their emotions and think before they act are less likely to present behavior problems. Youth who are trained to solve problems with others, give and receive feedback, and take on leadership roles are more likely to demonstrate positive social behaviors. Such benefits are associated with programs that are high quality and intentionally designed to bring about certain outcomes (Durlak, Weissberg, & Pachan, 2010; Greenberg et al., 2003; Zins, Weissberg, Wang, & Wahlberg, 2004). Sport programs designed merely to prevent crime by keeping at-risk youth "off the streets" rarely have the desired impact (Cutforth & Hellison, 1992).

Considering the demographics and social conditions in Belize, as well as the National Youth Development Policy (Youth Policy, 2013), we decided to focus our project on youth development using evidence-based best practices. While there is limited organization and coordination of youth sport in Belize, there is a significant number of national and city government programs, schools, and community organizations using sport to promote youth development. Using youth development as a central focus has allowed us to maximize the reach of BYSC by bringing together a wide variety of youth-serving agencies that offer sport programming.

Youth Development through Sport

Despite the widely held belief that "sport builds character," such benefits are not automatic. The culture of a youth sport program and the actions of a coach can just as easily teach negative lessons related to aggression, cheating, social exclusion, and winning at all costs (Theokas, 2009). Sport programs that claim to promote youth development must articulate how these principles and best practices are integrated (Petitpas et al., 2005). Sport-based youth development programs have great educational potential yet instead of feeling like "more school," they are active, exciting, and social (Peterson, 2013). Such programs can provide educational and developmental experiences that focus on social and emotional learning and life skill development (Hellison, 2011; Jacobs & Wright, 2014).

The teaching personal and social responsibility (TPSR) model (Hellison, 2011) is among the most well-established models for promoting positive youth development through sport (Petitpas et al., 2005). Its effectiveness has been demonstrated in physical education, after-school programs, and summer camps for more than 40 years (Hellison, 2011). The short-term goals of this model are for participants to develop respect for the rights and feelings of others, self-motivation, self-direction, and an ethic of caring. Practice sessions are structured to promote the importance of these responsibilities and practice them (e.g., resolving conflicts peacefully, setting goals, leading a group, and peer-coaching). The ultimate goal of TPSR is for youth to transfer these life skills to other settings such as school, home, and the community.

The literature indicates TPSR coaching strategies help youth to (a) develop an understanding of responsible behavior, (b) demonstrate these responsibilities in the program, and (c) apply TPSR values and life skills outside the program (Hellison, 2011; Hellison & Wright, 2003; Martinek & Lee, 2012). Outcomes include increases in youth leadership, responsibility, teamwork, and self-control (Hellison, 2011). Many studies indicate improvements in school performance as well as reductions in aggressive and antisocial behavior (Buckle & Walsh, 2013). TPSR is inclusive of ability and gender. It has proven successful in varied cultural contexts, including Spain, Portugal, Mexico, Brazil, Finland, New Zealand, and South Korea (Carbonell, 2012; Gordon, 2010; Jung & Wright, 2012; Martins, Rosado, Ferreira, & Biscaia, 2015).

Because TPSR is a field-tested approach to promoting youth development through sport, it was a cornerstone in the BYSC approach. This model provided a common set of values and objectives that aligned with local needs and the goals of the project. Moreover, because it can be applied with flexibility, it could be applied in a variety of contexts by individuals from different backgrounds, e.g., sport coaches, teachers, and youth workers. In sum, our conceptual framework integrated positive youth development, sport-based youth development, and social-emotional learning with a sport for diplomacy mission. We drew from the evidence-based best practices of the TPSR model (Hellison, 2011) to operationalize this framework and support our goal of promoting youth development and social change through sport.

Intentional Training

Research shows youth programs that are not intentionally designed or delivered with fidelity lack effectiveness (Durlak et al., 2010; Petitpas et al., 2005). Therefore, we invested heavily in training and developing capacity among local experts to enhance youth sport in Belize. Belize lacks a culture of professional development or certification for coaches. For example, there are no colleges or universities in Belize with degrees related to sport. Although physical education is required in the national curriculum, the country does not have the capacity to train and license professional physical education teachers. To obtain such training, individuals often travel to study to neighboring countries such as Mexico or Cuba.

In this environment, the majority of youth sport coaches have received no formal training, nor were they trained by coaches who did. Therefore, while our major emphasis was on youth development principles and the practical coaching strategies of TPSR, we did take the opportunity to address other foundational topics. For example, our training curriculum introduced background knowledge and practical strategies related to sport psychology, sport leadership, skill development, planning for instruction and coaching, as well as injury prevention.

Our intention in this project was not simply to deliver didactic training, but to develop capacity for the BYSC to continue and expand after the initial funding. To accomplish this, we trained administrators and coaches from many organizations. We also provided enhanced training to a group that was nominated by their peers to provide leadership. These individuals became certified BYSC trainers. The major training visits in this project are described below:

> **January 2014:** The first Belizean delegation traveled to the US. The delegation comprised five administrators representing national government departments, Belize City, and a nonprofit organization.

> **March 2014:** Six Americans traveled to Belize and provided coach training to 36 Belizeans representing approximately 10 different organizations.

> **November 2014:** Eight Belizean delegates, who had been trained in March 2014 and nominated by their peers as leaders in the BYSC, traveled to the US.

> **March 2015:** Six Americans traveled to Belize and provided training for 45 Belizean coaches, teachers, and youth workers. Belizean BYSC trainers served as cofacilitators with the American team.

Each of these major exchanges involved approximately 36 hours of training content delivered over four to five days. Training methods included lecture, discussion, model coaching sessions, peer coaching and practice opportunities, and debriefing sessions. Belizean delegates to the US went on site visits and participated in formal events to showcase the project. The November 2014 delegates being developed as BYSC trainers received advanced training on TPSR pedagogy, including methods to observe, assess, and give feedback on implementation fidelity. They also contributed to the plan for the March 2015 training that they would help to deliver.

Collective Impact

While training coaches to implement youth development principles and TPSR best practices has been a major focus, this is not a sufficient strategy to promote social change. For the BYSC to thrive requires participation and buy-in from several organizations. Only if a critical mass of organizations join and commit to pulling together could we hope to influence social change. Admittedly, this is a lofty goal, but the opportunity in Belize is unique and there are effective models for fostering collective impact that can be applied. Regarding the Belizean context, because it is such a small nation, building a coalition was a matter of practicality. Many Belizean youth-serving programs and agencies are small and lack the capacity to undertake significant training or strategic planning activities to improve their sport programs. However, a coalition comprising multiple organizations makes this possible. At the same time, because Belize is such a small nation, strategically including certain government offices and larger organizations in the coalition allows the BYSC to reach a substantial portion of youth. Finally, because Belize City has the highest concentration of youth, youth-serving programs, and criminal activity, it is a fulcrum for promoting youth development and social change.

Fostering collaborative efforts is vital to the success of any socially related initiative; however, often the success of individual efforts lacks the cohesiveness to reach a sustained level of effort and, as a result, becomes ineffective and inefficient and ultimately fails (Kania & Kramer, 2011). Any successful large-scale and sustainable social change initiative requires coordinated efforts from a number of different entities to shift focus from an isolated to a collective impact approach. Research by Kania and Kramer (2011) has found that most successful collective impact efforts include five main conditions: (a) common agenda, (b) shared measurement systems, (c) mutually reinforcing activities, (d) continuous communication, and (e) backbone support organizations (see Table 4-1).

Since 2013, the BYSC has been building partnerships and collaborations with national government, the Belize City government, nongovernmental, and higher education organizations. This is challenging because in Belize there is a culture of resistance to organizational collaboration related to sharing power (and credit), crossing sectors, perceived "territory," and political affiliations. However, collaboration is crucial because so many Belizean organizations lack the capacity to have community-level impact alone. Despite these obstacles, the BYSC has trained approximately 80 coaches, teachers, youth workers, and police officers representing approximately 20 different organizations.

Once the five conditions of collective impact have been established, three phases must be implemented to move an initiative forward (see Table 4-2). Many of the components for success associated with Phase I (Initiate Action) have already taken place in Belize. As our SportsUnited grant is nearing completion, we are taking on many of the Phase II (Organize for Impact) activities and helping the BYSC to move toward Phase III (Sustained Action and Impact).

Table 4-1. Five Conditions of Collective Impact

CONDITION	DEFINITION
Common Agenda	All participants have a shared vision for change including a common understanding of the problem and a joint approach to solving it through agreed upon actions.
Shared Measurement	Collecting data and measuring results consistently across all participants ensures efforts remain aligned and participants hold each other accountable.
Mutually Reinforcing Activities	Participant activities must be differentiated while still being coordinated through a mutually reinforcing plan of action.
Continuous Communication	Consistent and open communication is needed across the many players to build trust, assure mutual objectives, and create common motivation.
Backbone Support	Creating and managing collective impact requires a separate organization(s) with staff and a specific set of skills to serve as the backbone for the entire initiative and coordinate participating organizations and agencies.

Source: Adapted from Hanleybrown, Kania, & Kramer, 2012.

Table 4-2. Three Phases of Collective Impact

COMPONENTS FOR SUCCESS	PHASE II INITIATE ACTION	PHASE II ORGANIZE FOR IMPACT	PHASE III SUSTAINED ACTION AND IMPACT
Governance and Infrastructure	Identify champions, form groups	Create infrastructure	Facilitate and refine
Strategic Planning	Map the landscape, use data to make case	Create a common agenda	Support implementation
Community Involvement	Facilitate community outreach	Engage community and build public will	Continue engagement, conduct advocacy
Assessment and Improvement	Analyze baseline data to identify key issues and gaps	Establish shared metrics	Collect, track, and report progress

Source: Adapted from Hanleybrown et al., 2012.

Rigorous Evaluation

We are ardent believers in the value of rigorous program evaluation. Rather than limiting our evaluation to reporting outputs, e.g., the number of individuals trained, we have taken a comprehensive approach to evaluation and used data not only to document activities but to make improvements, inform next steps, and contribute to the academic literature. We have combined qualitative and quantitative methods to evaluate the BYSC (Patton, 2005). Throughout the project, we have administered training feedback surveys to assess the quality of the training, participant satisfaction, participant learning, and the relevance of the material. We have administered validated surveys to assess changes in trainees' self-efficacy for teaching personal and social skills. Individual and group interviews have been conducted to evaluate the training, assess learning, and understand barriers and facilitators to implementation. We have taken extensive field notes and documented the project with hundreds of photographs and several dozen hours of video. Supporting data sources include planning documents, training materials, meeting agendas, attendance and registration records, as well as communications with the U.S. State Department and the U.S. Embassy at Belmopan.

Our team has made use of program evaluation data throughout the project. We have used participant feedback during a training to make adjustments, such as including more hands-on practice or using examples from the local context to show the application of a strategy for conflict resolution. We have also used evaluation data to make larger changes in the direction of the program. For example, the framework of collective impact shared above was not part of our original proposal. However, as we came to understand the context, challenges, and opportunities better, we returned to the literature to find a more precise framework to guide a shared vision for the coalition. Another pragmatic use of formative evaluation relates to our funding obligations. Data have been used in quarterly reports to the SportsUnited program to provide updates on project milestones, problems encountered, lessons learned, etc.

This project also presents an opportunity to apply and develop best practices that can inform the academic literature. Beyond meeting the minimal expectation for evaluation, we have integrated this project with our scholarship. We use empirical findings to answer questions and address gaps in the literature related to sport for diplomacy, sport for development, and sport-based youth development. These lines of inquiry have resulted in conference presentations and manuscript submissions. We believe these pragmatic and academically oriented evaluation activities are valuable as they improve our delivery of the current program, enhance our ability to do similar work in the future, and inform others engaged in related work across the globe.

Accomplishments and Challenges

As our initial funding comes to an end, we are pleased with our progress. We have stayed close to our program plan and met our milestones with only slight deviations. We have encountered some difficulties meeting our output targets. For example, we have struggled to achieve the proposed level of gender balance. Opportunities for females to participate in sport lag behind opportunities for males in Belize. This is especially pronounced in sport leadership. We have worked hard to include female coaches and administrators, but these numbers are not equal. Also, because of the small scale of programs in Belize, the number of certified coaches and trainers is lower than originally projected. Regarding outputs and reach, we have achieved the following:

- hosted 13 delegates from Belize for training in the US and provided initial training for over 70 individuals in Belize;
- involved approximately 20 organizations from very small to very large in the BYSC with the majority sending multiple staffers for training;

- BYSC-trained coaches delivered programs to approximately 1,200 youth in summer 2014 and 1,500 in summer 2015; and

- during the 2015-2016 academic year, BYSC-trained coaches have worked with approximately 3,000 youth through school-based athletics, physical education, and after-school programs.

In claiming outputs, we acknowledge three points. First, while we are happy for the growth of this network and the reach we have seen thus far, we cannot account for the quality of implementation or impact in all cases. However, site visits and follow-up interviews confirm many of the BYSC-trained coaches have implemented content from their training to varying degrees. Second, in reporting the number of youth participants reached, we are aware there is redundancy. However, we do not necessarily see this as a problem. If an individual child participates in a BYSC-affiliated summer program two years in a row and during the school year receives consistent messages from her physical education teacher and sport director in school, as well as the youth workers she sees in an after-school program, this is a sign the collective impact model is working. Third, the reason our claims about program implementation and youth outcomes are tentative is that these factors are beyond the official scope of our funded project. The BYSC grant from SportsUnited funded a training program for coaches and administrators, so most of our data collection has focused on the training outcomes for these individuals.

Surveys, interviews, our own observations, and a site visit from the Public Affairs Section of the U.S. Embassy at Belmopan all reflect well on the quality and relevance of our training. Multiple data sources also indicate participant learning has been high. This applies to our initial coach training program as well as the advanced training offered to BYSC trainers. The BYSC trainers have demonstrated competency in delivering model lessons, planning, and co-facilitating training sessions, and achieving scores of 85% or higher on a performance-based assessment of their understanding of the TPSR model. In-depth interviews have revealed the BYSC trainers have had a transformative learning experience that has changed their perspective on the role of youth sport in supporting youth development and social change. This experience has also increased their confidence in their leadership abilities and their ability to advocate for youth sport in Belize (Wright, Jacobs, Ressler, & Jung, 2016).

As for supporting organizational change and laying the groundwork for sustainability, it has taken concerted effort but we are seeing progress. Through the first two years of the project, it appeared that without our direct involvement there was little followthrough or communication among local stakeholders. As explained above, we have seen many obstacles to collaboration across agencies and departments. However, by the third year of the grant, we have seen a clear increase in ownership and collaboration among local stakeholders. Some individuals and organizations have fallen away, but those who have stayed are becoming more invested. We have a clear leadership team representing multiple organizations. The YMCA of Belize has emerged as a backbone organization, taking a leadership role in convening stakeholders and pursuing sustainability funding from local sources. The level of ownership and capacity we see at this stage gives us cause for optimism. Our commitment is to maintain this relationship and continue to provide support, but our ultimate goal will be accomplished when the BYSC no longer relies on our assistance (Coalter, 2010). As Beer and Nohria (2000) have suggested, top-down change often poses more immediate economic upside (though often at the expense of sustainability); while bottom-up change often affords highers costs, but yields longer term results.

CONCLUSION

Interest in the use of sport for diplomacy has become increasingly widespread. The United Nations asserts, "Sport has a unique power to attract, mobilize and inspire," (United Nations, 2015, para 4). Accordingly, organizations around the world invest in programs that use sport as a vehicle for social change. Unfortunately, the quality of these programs varies and empirical literature on the topic is limited (Murray & Pigman, 2014). The BYSC is a unique sport-for-diplomacy program because of its emphasis on youth sport, intentional training, and capacity building. It has also taken a novel approach in applying positive youth development principles, the TPSR model, and the collective impact framework. Finally, we believe this case may be informative through its use of program evaluation to support program delivery and to develop best practices.

We have spent nearly three years working with local partners to develop the BYSC and make it a sustainable entity that can continue to promote youth development and social change in Belize. As this grant comes to an end, the BYSC appears to have the capacity and momentum to expand and implement programs that will produce measurable outcomes for youth participants. Without knowing what the future holds for the BYSC, we trust what has been developed and learned thus far demonstrates possibilities and stimulates thinking that may contribute to the rapidly expanding and important field of sport for diplomacy.

DISCUSSION QUESTIONS

1. Based on your opinion and what has been established in this book, define what is meant by the term *sport for diplomacy*. Based on your working definition, how does the BYSC fit within this field? Provide an explanation or rationale for your response.

2. What cultural, socioeconomic, and political factors should most influence the design and implementation of collective impact efforts in Belize? How and why might these factors influence progress?

3. Based on this chapter (and others presented in this text), describe and discuss the need for research and evaluation in sport for diplomacy programs.

4. How could the lessons learned from the BYSC project be used to shape or inform Belize's National Sport Policy?

5. What are the benefits of developing programs like the BYSC in partnership with local stakeholders as opposed to simply delivering an existing training program?

6. Given the high population of Belizeans under the age of 25, why you do think that initiatives that might improve youth sports in Belize go unfinished or unfunded?

7. You have recently been elected mayor of Belize City. Describe and overview two sport-based initiatives that would foster the development of youth sports in the city. Be sure to take into account the financial, economic, and social implications of these initiatives.

REFERENCES

Allport, G. W. (1954). *The nature of prejudice.* Cambridge, MA: Addison-Wesley.

Baker, R., Esherick, C., & Baker, P. (2011). Sport diplomacy: A program evaluation. Retrieved from http://citeseerx.ist.psu.edu/viewdoc/download?doi=10.1.1.471.1680&rep=rep1& type= pdf#page=29

Beer, M., & Nohria, N. (2000). Cracking the code of change. *Harvard Business Review, 78,* 133-141.

Belize National Sport Council. (2015). Ministry of education, culture, and sport. Retrieved from http://www.moe.gov.bz/index.php/sports-services

Breaking News Belize. (2015a, July 8). Belize will participate in Pan American games. Retrieved from http://www.breakingbelizenews.com/2015/07/08/belize-participate-pan-american-games/

Breaking News Belize. (2015b, August 4). Special Olympics athletes return with silver. Retrieved from http://www.breakingbelizenews.com/2015/08/04/special-olympics-athletes-return-silver/

Buckle, M. E., & Walsh, D. S. (2013). Teaching responsibility to gang-affiliated youths. *Journal of Physical Education, Recreation & Dance, 84,* 53-58.

Bureau of Educational and Cultural Affairs. (2013). Study of ECA's SportsUnited Programs. Retrieved from https://eca.state.gov/files/bureau/studyofsportsunited_report.pdf

Bureau of Educational and Cultural Affairs (2015). Retrieved from http://eca.state.gov/ programs-initiatives/sports-diplomacy

Carbonell, A. E. (2012). Applying the teaching personal and social responsibility model (TPSR) in Spanish schools context: Lesson learned. *Agora para la Educación Física y el Deporte, 14,* 178-196.

Catalano, R. F., Berglund, M. L., Ryan, J. A. M., Lonczak, H. S., & Hawkins, J. D. (2004). Positive youth development in the United States: Research findings on evaluations of positive youth development programs. *Annals of the American Academy of Political and Social Science, 591,* 98-124.

Channel 5 Belize. (2015a, October 29). Outgoing sports minister beats his chest over incomplete stadium. Retrieved from http://edition.channel5belize.com/archives/120630

Channel 5 Belize. (2015b, October 29). Mexican government funds multipurpose sports building at Marion Jones. Retrieved from http://edition.channel5belize.com/archives/120645

Chehabi, H. E. (2001). Sport diplomacy between the United States and Iran. *Diplomacy & State-craft, 12,* 89-106.

Coalter, F. (2010). The politics of sport-for-development: Limited focus programmes and broad gauge problems? *International Review for the Sociology of Sport, 45,* 295-314.

Crabbe, T. (2006). Reaching the 'hard to reach': Engagement, relationship building and social control in sport based social inclusion work. *International Journal of Sport Management and Marketing, 2,* 27-40.

Cutforth, N., & Hellison, D. (1992). Reflections on reflective teaching in a physical education teacher education methods course. *Physical Educator, 49*(3), 127-135.

Durlak, J. A., Weissberg, R. P., Pachan, M. (2010). A meta-analysis of after-school programs that seek to promote personal and social skills in children and adolescents. *American Journal of Community Psychology, 45,* 294-309.

Durlak, J. A., Weissberg, R. P., Dymnicki, A. B., Taylor, R. D., & Schellinger, K. B. (2011). The impact of enhancing students' social and emotional learning: A meta-analysis of school-based universal interventions. *Child Development, 82,* 405-432.

Gordon, B. (2010). An examination of the responsibility model in a New Zealand secondary school physical education program. *Journal of Teaching in Physical Education, 29,* 21-37.

Greenberg, M. T., Weissberg, R. P., O'Brien, M. U., Zins, J. E., Fredericks, L., Resnik, H., & Elias, M. J. (2003). Enhancing school-based prevention and youth development through coordinated social, emotional, and academic learning. *American Psychologist, 58*(6-7), 466-474.

Hanleybrown, F., Kania, J., & Kramer, M. R. (2012). Channeling change: Making collective impact work. *Stanford Social Innovation Review, 20,* 1-8.

Hartmann, D., & Kwauk, C. (2011). Sport and development: An overview, critique, and reconstruction. *Journal of Sport & Social Issues, 35,* 284-305.

Hellison, D. R. (2011). *Teaching personal and social responsibility through physical activity.* Champaign, IL: Human Kinetics.

Hellison, D. R., & Cutforth, N. J. (1997). Extended day programs for urban children and youth: From theory to practice. *Issues in Children's and Families Lives, 7,* 223-252.

Hellison, D., & Wright, P. (2003). Retention in an urban extended day program: A process-based assessment. *Journal of Teaching in Physical Education, 22,* 369-381.

International Platform on Sport and Development. (2015). About this platform. Retrieved from http://www.sportanddev.org/en/about_this_platform/

Jackson, S. J. (2013). The contested terrain of sport diplomacy in a globalizing world. *International Area Studies Review, 16,* 274-284.

Jacobs, J., & Wright, P. (2014). Social and emotional learning policies and physical education. *Strategies, 27*(6), 42-44.

Jung, J., & Wright, P. (2012). Application of Hellison's responsibility model in South Korea: A multiple case study of "at-risk" middle school students in physical education. *Agora para la Educación Física y el Deporte, 14,* 140-160.

Kania, J., & Kramer, M. (2011). Collective impact. Stanford Social Innovation Review, 1, 36-41.

Kidd, B. (2008). A new social movement: Sport for development and peace. *Sport in Society, 11,* 370-380.

Lawson, H. A. (2005). Empowering people, facilitating community development, and contributing to sustainable development: The social work of sport, exercise, and physical education programs. *Sport, Education and Society, 10,* 135-160.

Manzenreiter, W. (2008). Football diplomacy, post-colonialism and Japan's quest for normal state status. *Sport in Society, 11,* 414-428.

Martinek, T., & Lee, O. (2012). From community gyms to classrooms: A framework for values-transfer in schools. *Journal of Physical Education, Recreation & Dance, 83,* 33-51.

Martins, P., Rosado, A., Ferreira, V., & Biscaia, R. (2015). Examining the validity of the personal-social responsibility questionnaire among athletes. *Motriz: Revista de Educação Física, 21,* 321-328.

Ministry of Education, Youth, Sports, and Culture. (2015). Sports council. Retrieved from http://www.moe.gov.bz/index.php/sports-services

Murray, S., & Pigman, G. A. *(2014). Mapping the relationship between international sport and diplomacy. Sport* in Society, 17, 1098-1118.

Newman, J., & Dusenbury, L. (2015). Social and emotional learning (SEL): A framework for academic, social, and emotional success. In K. Bosworth (Ed.), *Prevention science in school settings* (pp. 287-306). New York, NY: Springer.

Patton, M. Q. (2005). *Qualitative research.* Hoboken, NJ: John Wiley & Sons, Inc.

Peterson, T. K. (2013). *Expanding minds and opportunities: Leveraging the power of afterschool and summer learning for student success.* Washington, DC: Collaborative Communications Group.

Petitpas, A. J., Cornelius, A. E., Van Raalte, J. L., & Jones, T. (2005). A framework for planning youth sport programs that foster psychosocial development. *The Sport Psychologist, 19,* 63-80.

Pigman, G. A., & Rofe, J. S. (2014). Special issue: Sport and diplomacy. *Sport in Society: Cultures, Commerce, Media, Politics, 17,* 1095-1223.

Pitts, B. G., & Stotlar, D. K. (2007). *Fundamentals of sport marketing* (3rd ed.). Morgantown, WV: Fitness Information Technology.

Ramos, A. (2014, September 16). Belize on Obama's list for drug trafficking. Retrieved from http://amandala.com.bz/news/belize-obamas-list-drug-trafficking/

Seven News Belize. (2013, April 3). Taking a swing at Belize's first national sports policy and strategic plan. Retrieved from http://www.7newsbelize.com/sstory.php?nid=25120

Spaaij, R. (2012). Beyond the playing field: experiences of sport, social capital, and integration among Somalis in Australia. *Ethnic and Racial Studies, 35,* 1519-1538.

Spaaij, R., & Jeanes, R. (2013). Education for social change? A Freirean critique of sport for development and peace. *Physical Education and Sport Pedagogy, 18,* 442-457.

Theokas, C. (2009). Youth sport participation-A view of the issues: Introduction to the special section. *Developmental Psychology, 45,* 303-306.

United Nations. (2015). Sport for development and peace: The UN system in action. Retrieved from www.un.org/wcm/content/site/sport/home/sport

United States Central Intelligence Agency. (2015). The World Factbook: Belize. Retrieved from https://www.cia.gov/library/publications/the-world-factbook/geos/bh.html

United States Overseas Security Advisory Council. (2013). Belize 2013 crime and safety report. Retrieved from https://www.osac.gov/pages/contentreportdetails.aspx?cid=14034

Wright, P. M., Jacobs, J. M., Ressler, J. D., & Jung, J. (2016). Teaching for transformative educational experience in a sport for development program. *Sport, Education and Society, 21,* 531-548.

Youth Policy. (2015). National youth development policy of Belize. Retrived from http://www.youthpolicy.org/national/Belize_2013_National_Youth_Development_Policy.pdf

Zins, J. E., Weissberg, R. P., Wang, M. C., & Walberg, H. J. (Eds.). (2004). *Building academic success on social and emotional learning: What does the research say?* New York, NY: Teachers College Press.

5

SPORT FOR HOPE IN HAITI: DISASTER DIPLOMACY OR DISASTER CAPITALISM?

SCOTT JEDLICKA

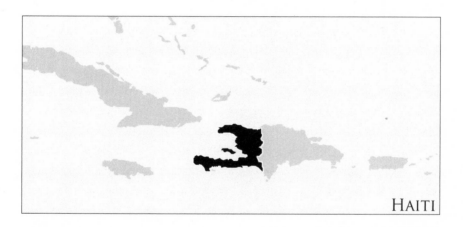

HAITI

ABSTRACT

In January 2010, a devastating earthquake struck Haiti, causing billions of dollars in damage, killing over 100,000 people, disfiguring several thousand more, and leaving nearly 2 million homeless (Bell, 2013). Two years later, the International Olympic Committee (IOC) began construction in the Haitian capital of Port-au-Prince of its second Sport for Hope Centre, a multifunctional sport facility that, once constructed, would provide educational and training opportunities for Haitian athletes of all abilities (IOC, 2012). The facility, a collaborative effort of the IOC, the Haitian government, the National Olympic Committee of Haiti (COH), and various other stakeholders, was completed in July

2014 at a cost of $18 million. This study considers Haiti's Sport for Hope Centre from two complementary perspectives on the relationship between catastrophic events and international relations: disaster diplomacy (Kelman, 2012) and disaster capitalism (Klein, 2007; Loewenstein, 2015). This analysis also reviews recent trends in international sport for development, especially efforts championed by the United Nations and the IOC, such as Olympic Agenda 2020. The case of Haiti's Sport for Hope Centre illustrates the conflicted nature of international sport for development initiatives and their relationship to broader political and economic trends, and calls for further reflection on the use of sport for political and quasipolitical purposes.

Keywords: Haiti, Sport for Hope, International Olympic Committee, sport for development, disaster diplomacy, disaster capitalism

SPORT FOR HOPE IN HAITI: DISASTER DIPLOMACY OR DISASTER CAPITALISM?

In 2012, the International Olympic Committee (IOC) began construction in the Haitian capital city of Port-au-Prince of its second Sport for Hope Centre, a multifunctional sport facility that, once completed, would provide educational and training opportunities for Haitian athletes of all abilities (IOC, 2012). The facility, a collaborative effort of the IOC, the Haitian government, the National Olympic Committee of Haiti (COH), and various other stakeholders, was completed in July 2014 at a cost of $18 million. The project is part of the IOC's Sport for Hope Program, the goal of which is to "provide young people and communities with opportunities to practice sport and be educated in the values of Olympism" (IOC, 2010a, p. 2). The first facility constructed as part of this development project was built in Lusaka, Zambia, in 2010. The Lusaka project and the Sport for Hope Program were praised in 2012 by United Nations (UN) Secretary-General Ban Ki-moon as examples of the power of sport to effect social change; two years later, Ban and IOC president Thomas Bach signed an historic agreement allowing for closer collaboration between the two organizations on sport for development initiatives (IOC, 2014a; UN Office on Sport for Development and Peace, 2012). The aggressiveness with which the IOC has pursued sport for development (i.e., using sport to stimulate socioeconomic improvements), in addition to its more traditional, self-ascribed duties as a global leader in sport development (i.e., increasing the quantity and quality of sport participation opportunities), is part of a larger strategic readjustment for the IOC encapsulated in Olympic Agenda 2020. This agenda, developed in 2014 and consisting of "20+20 recommendations to shape the future of the Olympic Movement," simultaneously emphasizes the need for more international cooperation in the use of sport for development purposes and the autonomy of the IOC to lead this effort (IOC, 2014b). Given the adoption of Olympic Agenda 2020 and the corresponding expansion of the IOC's province in international sport to include not just sport development but sport for development, the selection of Haiti as a beneficiary of the Sport for Hope program is not surprising.

By almost any measure, it would be difficult to describe Haiti as a sporting power-house. A Caribbean nation with a population of roughly 10.5 million and a gross domestic product per capita of just $1,794, Haiti arguably faces much more immediate and serious problems than a lack of success in sport (International Monetary Fund, 2015). However, this does not mean that Haiti cannot claim its share of sporting accomplishments. For instance, relative to teams from other Caribbean nations, Haitian soccer clubs have been some of the most consistent participants in the Caribbean Football Union (CFU) Club Champi-onship. Additionally, two different Haitian clubs have won the Confederation of North, Central American and Caribbean Association Football (CONCACAF) Champions League, equal to the number of champions hailing from the United States. On May 10, 2014, Cana-dian boxer Bermane Stiverne became the first Haitian-born World Boxing Council (WBC) heavyweight titleholder, defeating American Chris Arreola by technical knockout (Sim-mons, 2014). Despite these notable achievements, Haiti has not experienced much success in major international competitions nor developed a lucrative professional sport industry within its borders. The country's Olympic teams have won only two medals (a bronze in 1924 and a silver in 1928), and Haiti has never been represented at the Winter Olympics. The national soccer team has qualified for just a single World Cup (1974), losing all three of its matches by a combined 14-2 score. Haiti has produced a number of professional athletes, primarily in football, basketball, soccer, and boxing, but many of these athletes (like Sti-verne) represent or compete for teams in other countries. While Haiti is certainly not absent from the world of sport, its domestic and international sporting achievements have been relatively insignificant. Because of this general lack of sporting notoriety, the IOC's decision in 2010 to construct a state-of-the-art training facility in Haiti can be described in terms of the organization's long-standing role as a global leader in sport development. However, the IOC's decision cannot be fully explained or understood without acknowledging the broader crisis unfolding in Haiti at the time.

In January 2010, a devastating earthquake struck Haiti, causing billions of dollars in damage, killing over 100,000 people, disfiguring several thousand more, and leaving nearly 2 million homeless (Bell, 2013). The earthquake's immediate effects were exacerbated by the national government's inadequate response to the disaster. Despite an outpouring of international support in the days and months following the earthquake, initial recovery efforts were slow to develop and largely ineffective. Oxfam, an international NGO dedicated to addressing issues of poverty and social justice, was particularly critical of the Haitian gov-ernment's lack of urgency and inability to demonstrate "real political leadership" in rebuild-ing the island nation (Oxfam International, 2011). By 2012, the year the Sport for Hope Centre proposal was officially approved and construction began, over 500,000 Haitians remained homeless, many living in temporary structures and tents. Further, the slow rate of progress prompted increasingly pointed questions about the ways in which aid organiza-tions and the Haitian government were spending the billions of dollars donated to support recovery efforts (Robles, 2012). Amidst these struggles, the IOC championed its new facility as an important step forward in Haiti's rebuilding process. At a groundbreaking ceremony for the project, IOC member Mario Vázquez Raña said, "I am convinced that this effort will benefit young Haitian athletes, who are striving in the face of adversity" (IOC, 2012).

Haiti's Sport for Hope Centre was thus rationalized in terms of sport development, sport for development, and cooperative international disaster relief goals. The facility was ostensibly designed to promote elite as well as mass sport participation in Haiti, and was also characterized as an integral part of the earthquake recovery effort. These rationales, as well as the circumstances in which they were deployed, can in turn be explained in terms of two related but distinct perspectives on the relationship between natural (or manmade) disasters and international politics: *disaster diplomacy* (Kelman, 2012), which examines the potential for catastrophic events to foster cooperation or conflict among international actors, and *disaster capitalism* (Giardina & Cole, 2012; Klein, 2007), a highly critical view of the political opportunism exhibited by governments in implementing unpopular domestic and foreign policies in the wake of such events. On one hand, Haiti's new facility and the IOC's Sports for Hope program in general can be considered examples of sport's semiotic power to inspire, uplift, and unify, even in the face of overwhelming tragedy. The eagerness of the usually apolitical IOC to work with governments and intergovernmental organizations, especially through Olympic Agenda 2020, could signal a renewed effort to engage sport for meaningful development. On the other hand, the Haitian government's prioritization of sport over more fundamental societal needs might indicate an overestimation of sport's importance to the developing world, and more alarmingly, a willingness of governments and sport organizations to exploit beliefs about sport for profit. This is especially salient considering the persistent questions regarding how disaster relief funds were spent and the fact that many Haitians still (in 2015) live without adequate shelter or sanitation.

REDEFINING THE IOC'S POLITICAL ROLE: SPORT FOR HOPE AND OLYMPIC AGENDA 2020

The IOC has had a longstanding interest in and commitment to its self-perceived role as an international diplomatic actor, even as it has often maintained—particularly under the leadership of Avery Brundage—a staunch devotion to the idea that Olympic sport is "apolitical" (Beacom, 2012; Guttmann, 1984). Indeed, the IOC's simultaneous insistence on its political relevance and separateness is today codified in its mission statement, which defines the IOC's role as leader of the Olympic movement in terms of "cooperat(ing) with the competent public or private organisations and authorities in the endeavour *to place sport at the service of humanity and thereby to promote peace"* as well as "tak(ing) action to strengthen the unity of the Olympic Movement, *to protect its independence and to preserve the autonomy of sport"* (IOC, 2015a, p. 18, emphasis added). In simpler terms, Olympic sport's effectiveness at promoting peace is believed to be contingent upon the Olympic movement remaining free from political interference; if sport is politicized—historically understood as any effort to undermine the IOC's "supreme authority and leadership"—Olympic sport can no longer fulfill its humanitarian objectives (IOC, 2015a, p. 17).

The IOC's interpretation of its political neutrality (or perhaps political transcendence) subtly but meaningfully shifted in September 2014, when IOC President Thomas Bach explicitly dispelled the notion that a bright line exists between sport and politics, saying,

> In the past, some have said that sport has nothing to do with politics, or they have said that sport has nothing to do with money or business. And this is just an attitude which is wrong and which we cannot afford anymore. (Abrahamson, 2014)

Bach's comment came less than six months after the landmark agreement between the UN and the IOC that ostensibly laid the foundation for closer collaboration between the two organizations, and just three months after the opening of Haiti's Sport for Hope Center in Port-au-Prince. Uttered during a speech at the Asian Games in Incheon, South Korea (UN Secretary-General Ban's native country), this unprecedented assertion of sport's political relevance by a leader of the Olympic movement marked a distinct change in tone for the IOC and likely signaled its shifting strategic priorities in advance of its adoption of Olympic Agenda 2020.

One of the most significant reasons for the IOC's effort to reorient itself was (and is) the growing public opposition to the economic and environmental impacts of the Olympics. While the financial, social, and environmental costs of Olympic events have been subject to criticism for decades, the declining number of bidding host cities (especially for the 2022 Winter Olympics, ultimately awarded in 2015 to Beijing) and the astronomical cost over-runs at the 2014 Sochi Winter Olympics intensified the perception that hosting the Olympics makes little economic sense for cities (Kilgore, 2015; Zimbalist, 2015). Collectively, a closer relationship with the UN, Bach's remarks acknowledging sport's connection to political matters, as well as the development of programs and policies like Olympic Agenda 2020 and Sport for Hope, indicate the IOC's changing understanding of its political role in response to growing public disapproval. No longer making unequivocal claims about political separateness, the IOC has redefined its role in global politics, placing a greater emphasis on the use of sport to meet local and international development objectives.

OLYMPIC AGENDA 2020

On December 7, 2014, in a speech marking the IOC's adoption of Olympic Agenda 2020, IOC President Bach reiterated his remarks from three months prior, emphasizing the need for the organization to adapt to a changing world as well as noting the unsustainability of the IOC's traditional attitude toward sport's relationship with politics and society (IOC, 2014b). Part of this ongoing adjustment process includes closer collaboration with the UN, nongovernmental organizations (NGOs), and national governments, relationships the IOC has traditionally avoided for fear of becoming entangled in or tainted by political issues. However, embedded in this rhetoric of greater international cooperation regarding the use of sport for development and maintaining the relevance of Olympic principles in a changing society is a distinct reaffirmation of the IOC's autonomy and preeminence in global sport (IOC, 2014b). These claims to autonomy, while seemingly redundant to those familiar with the principles and policies of the Olympic movement, this time carried new legal force: on October 16, 2014, the UN adopted Resolution A/69/L.5, which, among other things, "supports the independence and autonomy of sport as well as the mission of the International Olympic Committee in leading the Olympic movement" (UN General Assembly, 2014, p. 5). As the IOC rolled out Olympic Agenda 2020, it is important to note that this considerable overhaul to the IOC's priorities can be interpreted as somewhat of a quid pro quo in which the IOC agreed to lend its significant expertise, brand equity, and financial clout to the UN's sport-for-development initiatives in exchange for explicit guarantees regarding its leadership status in world sport. Using this reading, it remains unclear whether Olympic Agenda 2020 is a genuine reassessment of the IOC's roles in sport development and sport for development or simply a politically expedient measure, a way for the Olympic movement to consolidate power and create political alliances in the face of increased public scrutiny.

The content of Olympic Agenda 2020 is thus potentially shaped by the dual purposes of expanding and revising the Olympic movement's mission while ensuring that the IOC retains its position of power within international sport. This is significant for this study because one of the 40 recommendations composing Olympic Agenda 2020 involves the Sport for Hope program. Recommendation 24 calls on the IOC to "evaluate the Sport for Hope progamme" and specifically for

> The IOC to evaluate the success and impacts of the Sport for Hope programme over the next two to three years and, in the meantime, limit the programme to the two existing centres in Haiti and Zambia.

> The IOC to develop a sustainable operational model for the two existing Sport for Hope centres and invite other NGOs to contribute their particular areas of expertise, with the goal of having the centres become self-sufficient, managed and operated by another entity, and no longer reliant on the direct heavy investment and support of the IOC.

> The IOC to define further strategy of investment in locally adapted grass-roots sport facilities, building on the experience and lessons learned from the Olympafrica model (IOC, 2014b, p. 19).

The key components of this recommendation essentially call for an embargo on any further construction of Sport for Hope facilities and an effort to divest the IOC of what are implied to be burdensome resource commitments currently required by the existing centers; aside from the third item (a generic call for further study), it does not seem as though the Sport for Hope program is highly prioritized as part of Olympic Agenda 2020. This is an interesting contradiction given the glowing statements and noble rationales used to justify the construction of the Zambian and Haitian Sport for Hope facilities.

SPORT FOR HOPE—LUSAKA, ZAMBIA

The IOC's Sport for Hope program was initiated in 2010 during Jacques Rogge's presidency. The program's original conception envisioned the construction of multi-use sport facilities in the developing world. These centers would serve an array of purposes, including the provision of training opportunities and health services as well as the creation of a space for community gatherings and educational programs. As the program's name suggests, its overarching objective was value-driven, motivated by "the belief and experience that sport and its related facets... have the power to bring hope and development" (IOC, 2010a, p. 2).

The first Sport for Hope center (officially the Olympic Youth Development Center, or OYDC) opened in 2010 in Lusaka, Zambia. Originally designed to include spaces for athletics, field hockey, soccer, boxing, and a number of indoor sports such as basketball, handball, tennis, and volleyball, the center was also intended to "provide community development services and Olympic education, covering girls' empowerment, civic education and health services on HIV & AIDS, malaria and other health issues" (IOC, 2010a, p. 4). While the land for the project was gifted by the Zambian government, private organizations largely controlled the development effort; the IOC and several international sport federations (IFs) were responsible for managing the facility's construction and providing technical advice, and the center is currently operated by the National Olympic Committee (NOC) of Zambia (IOC, 2010b). Within a few years, the good feelings and optimism associated with the OYDC were becoming more difficult to sustain. In 2013, an anonymous letter posted on the Zambian Watchdog (an investigative journalism website) advanced allegations of financial corruption and sexual misconduct by the center's director, Clement Chileshe (Zambian Watchdog, 2013). The letter's author claimed that Chileshe, who was active in many sport for development efforts in Zambia at the time, was misappropriating funds from the IOC and other international sport organizations as well as making unwanted advances to female staff members. In contrast to these allegations, proponents of the Sport for Hope project claimed success in 2014 when a 16-year-old Zambian sprinter who trained at the Sport for Hope facility won a gold medal in the 100 meters at the Summer Youth Olympic Games in Nanjing, China (Butler, 2014b).

Despite this notable achievement as well as several vague allusions to the center's positive social impact since its completion, there is scarce evidence that the OYDC in Lusaka is actually serving the purposes for which it was created. The lack of any measurable effects is made all the more concerning by the corruption charges as well as the fact that the OYDC's construction involved the transfer of public wealth (i.e., the site for the facility) into private hands—a trend that appears to be continuing as the Zambian government considers whether to transfer control of the country's sport policymaking away from the government-run Sports Council of Zambia (SCZ) to the Zambian NOC (*Times of Zambia,* 2015). Regardless of whether these were intended consequences of the Sport for Hope initiative in Zambia, the program's pilot project illustrates both the difficulties associated with implementation and the (sometimes large) gap between rhetoric and reality when it comes to sport for development.

Both the initial Sport for Hope facility in Zambia and the more comprehensive Olympic Agenda 2020 signaled an adjustment of the IOC's priorities and indicated the organization's new understanding of its position vis-à-vis international relations. No longer content (or perhaps able) to adopt a laissez-faire approach to "politics," the IOC's move toward direct investment in sport for development and closer collaboration with governments and other international organizations reflects the two major normative tenets of Olympic Agenda 2020 and the IOC-UN agreement: that the IOC ought to use its significant resources to facilitate the use of sport for political (mostly development) objectives, and that the IOC's position as the preeminent international sport organization ought to be preserved. Arguably, the Sport for Hope program served as a testing ground for the ideas that were ultimately codified in Olympic Agenda 2020. While the Lusaka facility continues to be championed as a success story, the second Sport for Hope center constructed in Haiti is perhaps more revealing of the IOC's overall strategy in developing these programs. Additionally, the circumstances surrounding the Haiti facility's construction and operation might also explain why Sport for Hope is relegated to a position of apparent unimportance in Olympic Agenda 2020.

REBUILDING IN THE WAKE OF DISASTER: HAITI'S SPORT FOR HOPE CENTRE

The earthquake that occurred in Haiti on January 12, 2010, lasted only 35 seconds, yet its effects persist to this day. Nearly 1.9 million Haitians (more people than live in the state of Nebraska) lost their homes and belongings in the earthquake, surviving in tent shelters and shantytowns without adequate nutrition or sanitation (Bell, 2013). In the days and weeks following the disasters, medical services were overwhelmed—with morgues quickly reaching capacity, corpses lined the streets, while the wounded gathered in hospitals that were woefully undersupplied and understaffed (Charles, Clark, & Robles, 2010). By October 2010, the nation was facing a cholera outbreak, the first time the disease had been diagnosed in Haiti in nearly 100 years. A UN independent panel concluded that the disease had likely been introduced into Haiti by a foreign relief worker and had quickly spread due to the lack of hygienic water and waste management systems (UN, 2010). This finding encapsulates the duality of post-quake international intervention in Haiti. The international effort to provide assistance in the wake of the earthquake was viewed as both unprecedented (in terms of dollars pledged) and necessary given the Haitian government's inability to effectively manage the situation. However, as the recovery effort stretched from months into years with only incremental progress, the nature, effectiveness, and necessity of these international support measures (including the ways in which funding was spent by international organizations and the local government) were more frequently called into question.

INTERNATIONAL AID (AND OPPORTUNISM)

The outpouring of international support for Haiti following the earthquake was immense. National governments, NGOs, and for-profit corporations all pledged direct support in the

form of money, relief workers, and supplies, and many also facilitated individual donations to the relief efforts. However, the vast sums being shuffled from one organization to
another in the name of humanitarian aid for Haiti did not always translate into meaningful
recovery for Haitians. While the UN's Office for the Coordination of Humanitarian Affairs
(UNOCHA) reports that Haiti has received roughly $3.5 billion since 2010 in humanitarian
aid (with another approximately $925 million pledged but not committed), nearly 80,000
people were still living in makeshift housing in January 2015 (Charles, 2015; UNOCHA,
2015). Where has the money gone, or more specifically, why has it not had the intended
effect? Two explanations seem most prevalent among those who are willing to pose the
question. One involves the nature of the international aid "industry" and the other involves
an historical understanding of Haiti's relationship with the West.

When money is committed to humanitarian aid efforts, it is not simply a matter of one
government or international NGO depositing the sum into the accounts of the affected
national government or a local NGO. The process often involves complex interactions
among a number of organizations that are responsible for channeling the money into the
appropriate hands. As the number of interactions grows and as money is funneled through
organization after organization, the direct impact of the committed financial support is
reduced by the time it finally reaches its intended recipients. This is particularly true when
it comes to awarding contracts for construction projects and other initiatives, which can
create jobs and stimulate the local economy in addition to having a positive impact on the
community. In the case of Haiti, one organization in particular that has received a great deal
of criticism for its role in this process is the United States Agency for International Development (USAID). Within the first 18 months following the earthquake, it was reported that
only 2.5% of humanitarian aid funds had been distributed to Haitian companies and that
USAID had not awarded any business to Haitian contractors (Weisbrot, 2011). The housing
project overseen by USAID was approved in 2013 and was originally intended to construct
15,000 houses at a cost of $53 million; two years later, over $90 million had been spent
and only 2,600 homes had been built. On top of this, one estimate suggests that for every
dollar distributed by USAID for relief projects in Haiti, less than one cent went to Haitian
organizations (Johnston, 2015a, 2015b). While these reports imply USAID malfeasance,
local governments are not and should not be immune from scrutiny; for instance, a recent
study of disaster relief in Bulgaria suggested that an influx of international relief funds was
positively correlated with corrupt behavior in municipal government (Nikolova & Marinov,
2015). Other researchers contend that the lion's share of corruption is not governmental,
but occurs within the large bureaucracies of the international aid industry (Hancock, 1989).
Whether fiscal mismanagement is simply inherent to the humanitarian aid process or indic-
ative of something slightly more sinister, it is relatively clear that the relief funds committed
to Haiti have not resulted in the desired effects.

A more general explanation for why disaster relief in Haiti has been inefficient and ineffective involves an understanding of Haiti's past. Colonized first by the Spanish and then
the French (as well as enduring a brief period of U.S. occupation), populated by natives,

colonists, and slaves, Haitian society has developed over time into an amalgam of European and Caribbean cultural elements (Dayan, 1995). Politically, Haiti has been an independent nation since the early nineteenth century, though it has struggled to achieve domestic political stability. Its agriculture-based economy combined with its geographical position makes for an inconsistent economic environment as well. These factors combine to produce the situation, described by Haitian author Jean-Claude Martineau, in which "Haiti's last name [is] 'the poorest country in the Western Hemisphere.'" A more recent analysis simply describes Haiti as "collateral damage in the global political economy" (Bell, 2013, p. 31). Viewed through this critical lens, the international response to the earthquake in Haiti (especially the misuse of relief funds) is characterized as a continuation of an ongoing exploitative process in which white, Western hegemony continues to exert its mostly negative influence over Haiti and countries like it (Dantò, 2015).

This tension surrounding international relief efforts—their status as both necessary and unwanted—informs the context in which the IOC's Sport for Hope Centre was visualized and ultimately realized. Like other relief efforts, the Sport for Hope program (as noted previously) was rationalized at least partially in terms of disaster relief and harnessing the "power of sport" for desirable social ends. While the earthquake certainly did no favors for Haiti's already-lacking sport infrastructure, the IOC's decision to construct the Sport for Hope Centre (and the Haitian government's corresponding decision to accept this offer) was arguably motivated by more than simply a benevolent desire to assist in Haiti's recovery through the use of sport.

SPORT FOR HOPE COMES TO HAITI

In October 2010, shortly after the Zambian OYDC was completed and around the same time the cholera outbreak was beginning in northern Haiti, the IOC announced its intention to construct a second Sport for Hope Centre in Haiti. IOC spokesman Mark Adams said,

> One of the main reasons we chose Haiti was because of the recent earthquake there, so it was decided that would be a good place to take our help and try to take sport development to the people of Haiti. Straight humanitarian aid is always welcome, but I think the IOC felt that what we could do best is to offer the help and expertise that we have, which is obviously the sporting domain. (Associated Press, 2010)

Adams also added that the center would provide "a more lasting legacy," presumably for the IOC. The IOC contracted with CSA Group, a firm based in Miami, Florida, to manage the project, which involved selecting a general contractor to perform the actual construction of the facility as well as overseeing the project's schedule, budget, and quality (CSA Group, 2012). U.S.-based General Electric provided the lighting system, and the multinational corporation Mondo along with the International Association of Athletics Federations (IAAF) supplied the materials for the athletics track (General Electric, 2014; IAAF, 2014). However, similar to many disaster-relief contracts, it is difficult to know how much of the estimated $18 million the facility eventually cost was allocated to CSA Group or to know which other firms were subcontracted to complete the center's construction. As in Zambia, the national government authorized the use of the land for the facility.

When the center opened in July 2014, the similarities to Zambia's OYDC were evident. The complex comprises two large indoor training facilities, an indoor competition facility with a seating capacity of 2,500 and several outdoor playfields. Additionally, the center is also intended to house educational, social, and cultural development programs (Butler, 2014a). Despite the glowing remarks from IOC President Thomas Bach and Haitian President Michel Martelly about the center's potential positive effects, a 2015 Canadian Broadcasting Corporation report painted a different picture, one in which the parking lot of the facility sat empty and in which facility usage is restricted to wealthy children bused in from other parts of the country (Thomson, 2015). The CBC report and others note that the Sport for Hope Centre is built beneath the hillside shantytown of Canaan, where residents live in makeshift shelters without running water or electricity.

On the first anniversary of the center's opening, an IOC report described several hundred children learning to play table tennis, as well as coaching programs introducing the sports of field hockey and rugby to Haitian coaches (IOC, 2015b). While it is still too soon to tell whether Haiti will be able to claim an Olympic medalist as Zambia now does, another similarity between the two facilities is also apparent. In both cases, there seems to be very little available evidence of the centers' impacts beyond sport; what evidence does exist suggests that while these projects may be helping to develop elite athletes and increase sport participation to some degree in their respective countries, other development effects have yet to be realized.

DISASTER DIPLOMACY AND DISASTER CAPITALISM: POLITICS IN TIMES OF CRISIS

The political relevance of natural or human-caused catastrophic events has not received a great deal of scholarly attention. The research that has been conducted generally aligns with one of two distinct perspectives. *Disaster diplomacy* is rooted in a political science tradition, investigating "how and why disaster-related activities do and do not induce cooperation amongst enemies" (Kelman, 2012, p. 13). While not explicitly associated with disaster diplomacy as defined by Kelman, the study of humanitarian NGOs associated with disaster relief also provides some insight into the relationship between catastrophic events and international politics (Krause, 2014; Middleton & O'Keefe, 1998) *Disaster capitalism* is a perspective not specifically developed by academics, but rather by journalists who through their work have experienced first-hand the social and political effects of crisis events (Klein, 2007; Loewenstein, 2015). Disaster capitalism particularly focuses on the ways in which large-scale disasters are leveraged for unpopular (and potentially calamitous) political changes, such as the privatization of public services and the eradication of domestic barriers to foreign investment. The IOC's decision to construct a Sport for Hope Centre in Port-au-Prince can be explained and understood in terms of each of these perspectives.

SPORT FOR HOPE AS DISASTER DIPLOMACY

The idea that a program like the IOC's Sport for Hope initiative could serve a diplomatic function is aligned with the concept of disaster diplomacy, particularly with what Kelman (2012) calls *success pathways*. Success pathways are diplomatic strategies that states can employ to create stronger diplomatic relationships with other states through addressing disaster-related issues—in other words, using a disaster to successfully create or reaffirm existing international relationships. There is not space here to describe and explain each strategy, but in general, these approaches involve patience, multiple points of mutually desired contact between the states involved, appeals to objectivity (such as scientific evidence) and the use of symbols. When diplomatic efforts surrounding a disaster exhibit these elements, it is much more likely that new or better diplomatic relations will result. Though these success pathways are derived from cases involving state-to-state interaction, their underlying logic might be usefully abstracted and applied to other sorts of international relationships. Indeed, the prevalence and importance of nonstate actors in administering disaster relief cannot be overlooked, especially given the astronomical sums committed to recovery efforts in Haiti (Brattberg & Sundelius, 2011).

The primary actors involved in the Sport for Hope program in Haiti were not both states, but rather a state (Haiti) and an NGO (the IOC). In this sense, the overarching goal (from a disaster diplomacy standpoint) may not have been to establish good working relations, but simply for both parties to obtain some benefit from the relationship. For the IOC, the Sport for Hope facility was clearly aligned with its broader strategic shift toward emphasizing sport for development projects; for Haiti, the Sport for Hope facility may have been an opportunity to stimulate a long-dormant national sport program or simply to (as the name of the program suggests) provide some measure of optimism to a weary populace. Given these possibilities, the most salient disaster diplomacy concepts (i.e., success pathways) for analyzing the Sport for Hope program in Haiti are the themes (identified above) of mutuality and symbolism.

The idea that successful disaster diplomacy involves a high degree of mutuality simply means that the relationship must utilize multiple points of contact between the affected stakeholders. In a more traditional diplomatic relationship, this might mean contact not only between each state's respective ambassadors, but also between heads of state, members of relevant national agencies, and even nonstate actors and representatives. Although the Haitian government ceded the land for the Sport for Hope project and approved the construction, it is not clear whether or to what extent local community members in Port-au-Prince were consulted, or whether they even wanted the facility; available reports indicate only that the project was a partnership among the IOC, private investors and vendors, and the national government. Moreover, there appears to be a distinct lack of local involvement in the actual construction of the facility, and it is not evident that Haiti's Olympic

Committee (COH) had a great deal of input on the project either, aside from being tasked with its operation once it was completed. This suggests that the high degree of mutuality necessary to make this a successful diplomatic endeavor was not present. Though the most powerful stakeholders (the government and the IOC) approved of the project, its long-term success will likely depend on individuals and groups—especially at the local level—who were seemingly not consulted in the planning stages. Further, it is unclear whether the levels of comprehensive stakeholder engagement that would make this project an example of successful disaster diplomacy can or will be obtained.

The power of symbolic action also influences the success of disaster diplomacy. Kelman (2012) defines this concept in terms of how the actions of states are interpreted by other states—for instance, when a state accepts unnecessary disaster aid in order to signal its commitment to a deeper relationship with a donor state. Though the Sport for Hope program did not involve such a scenario, the more essential point regarding symbolism still applies to this case. Most notably, the entire project was to some extent rationalized in terms of its symbolic power. By offering to construct the facility, the IOC signaled its commitment to sport for development; by accepting the facility, Haiti signaled its commitment to sport and to sport's alleged power to inspire and uplift. However, the actions of the IOC and the Haitian government can also be interpreted less optimistically. While proponents of the Sport for Hope Centre see a meaningful symbol of a renewed Haiti, others—particularly many Haitians—may see yet another unwanted (Western) intervention in a poor island nation that benefits a select few but symbolizes nothing more than an opportunity cost or social burden for the remainder of the population.

Emphasizing these two elements of successful disaster diplomacy illustrates not only how the Sport for Hope Centre in Haiti may have fallen short of its stated development goals, but also that the opportunity exists for these sorts of sport-based projects to produce mutually desirable effects for both the IOC and the host country. Applying the concepts of successful disaster diplomacy to sport for development may be a way for sport organizations and governments to more effectively realize the potential of sport to produce positive individual and social effects. In Haiti's case, a more comprehensive consultation of local populations and greater sensitivity to the possible symbolic interpretations of the Sport for Hope Centre may have influenced how (or whether) the IOC chose to use the earthquake as an opportunity to implement this program.

SPORT FOR HOPE AS DISASTER CAPITALISM

In her 2007 book *The Shock Doctrine,* Naomi Klein defined disaster capitalism as "orchestrated raids on the public sphere in the wake of catastrophic events, combined with the treatment of disasters as exciting market opportunities" (p. 6). One of Klein's central theses is that deregulated, free market economic theories (such as those advocated by Milton Friedman) cannot be completely applied in democratic political systems—forcing a society comprising citizens with divergent and conflicting interests to perfectly adhere to the tenets of an economic model is simply unrealistic. Recounting the rise of global capitalism and neoliberalism since the 1970s, she points out that the radical implementation of free market systems in countries where they had not previously existed was consistently linked to natural or man-made disasters. In other words, the spread of globalization was and is not a natural process, but an exploitation of catastrophes (and the concomitant disarray and panic associated with these events) by powerful groups to implement free market policies that would otherwise have been politically impossible.

Certainly, the construction of the Sport for Hope Centre in Port-au-Prince does not rise to the level of radical economic policy changes. However, much like disaster diplomacy, the more general logic that informs the disaster capitalism perspective can be applied to the Sport for Hope case as well. To assess whether Haiti's Sport for Hope Centre is an example of disaster capitalism in action, it may be helpful to first consider a counterfactual scenario in which the earthquake never took place. In other words, would the IOC and Haiti have both decided to build the facility in the absence of a natural disaster? From Haiti's perspective, it seems likely that the national government would still have agreed to the project even without the earthquake, though it may have faced stiffer public opposition since citizens would not have been focused on more immediate and dire concerns associated with earthquake recovery; questions regarding the project's opportunity costs as well as equality of access to the completed facility may have been more forcefully raised and more thoroughly considered in a less calamitous context.

From the IOC's perspective, the probable outcome is less apparent. On one hand, even without the earthquake, Haiti would have still been an attractive candidate for a Sport for Hope facility. The country's high poverty levels and lack of a strong sporting tradition would have been a good fit for the stated objectives of the Sport for Hope program. On the other hand, the IOC's initial selection of Haiti as the site for the second Sport for Hope facility was explained almost entirely in terms of earthquake recovery, and there is little evidence to suggest one way or another that Haiti was under consideration prior to the disaster.

A second consideration in determining whether the IOC's efforts in Haiti can be called disaster capitalism is to, in simple terms, follow the money. Disaster capitalism is typically identified by the privatization of state services and an influx of foreign investment. Again, while the Sport for Hope Centre does not represent any sweeping change to national economic policy, the project still arguably features elements that might be associated with disaster capitalism. For instance, the fact that publicly controlled land was gifted to a private, international organization like the IOC (rather than developed for the same use by the government) may be an example of the sort of privatization typically seen during instances of disaster capitalism. Correspondingly, the facility is operated by an ostensibly private organization (the COH). The fact that the construction itself involved foreign and multinational (as opposed to local) organizations and corporations may also support the disaster capitalism characterization, in the sense that the project, especially in the wake of the earthquake, was viewed by these foreign organizations as an opportunity for positive publicity or financial profit.

The notion that the Sport for Hope Centre in Haiti can be characterized as disaster capitalism does not necessarily suggest that the project was motivated by malicious or exploitative intentions. However, it does suggest that the creation of the facility and its continued operation might be viewed through this lens. In other words, even if the IOC, the COH, the Haitian government, and other stakeholders did not willfully intend to take control of public resources for private gain or use the earthquake as an excuse to share in the billions of dollars flowing through Haiti in the name of disaster recovery, this is a possible (and perhaps likely) interpretation of their motives. As the IOC and other international sport organizations continue to collaborate with the public and nonprofit sectors in using sport for development purposes, cases like Haiti indicate the potential for such efforts to be read as exploitative.

SPORT FOR INTERNATIONAL DEVELOPMENT: WHO BENEFITS?

The IOC is clearly committed to sport for development as a strategic priority. The various components of Olympic Agenda 2020 spell this out in great detail and the apparent good feelings between IOC and UN leaders provide ample support for this assertion. In many ways, this marks a significant inflection point in the IOC's history. Up until recently, the Olympic movement was more or less content to claim that sport (and the Olympics in particular) was a sufficient condition for achieving the movement's humanitarian objectives; so long as athletes from around the world could compete peacefully, the Olympic movement could theoretically fulfill its goals. By endeavoring to work more closely with national governments and other international organizations, the IOC has thoroughly debunked that belief. The case of Haiti's Sport for Hope Centre provides some clues as to how the IOC's newfound willingness to engage in global politics will affect international sport and international relations.

Regardless of whether disaster diplomacy or disaster capitalism is employed as the explanatory framework, the Sport for Hope project in Haiti could have been better managed. While the most powerful actors said and did all of the right things, the stark reality of the situation that persists in Haiti today suggests that the facility's construction was ill-timed and perhaps ill-conceived. Given the concerns about the misallocation of disaster relief funds by humanitarian organizations even prior to the facility's groundbreaking, the IOC's construction of an $18 million facility in the shadow of a tent village seems, at best, tone deaf. In the future, efforts to construct such facilities might employ some of the success pathways for disaster diplomacy discussed above while being cognizant of the broader global forces that inform and perpetuate disaster capitalism. If sport is to inspire hope and foster social development, programs like Sport for Hope must solicit input from the people who stand to obtain these benefits and who are most directly affected by the existence of the facilities and programs designed to provide them. This is especially true if these programs are to take on the added burden of assisting in disaster recovery efforts.

Perhaps this necessary level of commitment is why the Sport for Hope program is so heavily deemphasized in Olympic Agenda 2020. The requirements for effectively implementing such a program, coupled with the arguably more pressing concerns regarding the economic and environmental sustainability of the Olympic festivals, may simply be too costly for the IOC to maintain. However, this possibility as to why the Sport for Hope program is currently "under evaluation" underscores the often unacknowledged gulf between ideas and action in sport for development. Championing sport for development makes good sense for the IOC given its stated mission and values as well as its aspirations to political relevance. The more important question is whether the IOC can or should follow through on these commitments even when they present a financial burden. In Haiti, the Sport for Hope Centre is built and ready to fulfill the idealistic promises its creators made for it. It remains to be seen whether the IOC will continue to invest in programs like Sport for Hope and more importantly, the calculus it will employ in making that decision.

DISCUSSION QUESTIONS

1. To what extent can sport development objectives (e.g., increasing sport participation and developing elite athletes) and sport for development objectives (e.g., using sport for promoting public health and social inclusion) be effectively pursued simultaneously in a program like Sport for Hope?

2. How will the IOC's willingness to work more closely with national governments and international NGOs influence the use of sport as a tool of global diplomacy and development?

3. Which of the two theoretical perspectives introduced in the case—disaster diplomacy and disaster capitalism—best explains the IOC's efforts in Haiti? Why?

4. Would Haiti (and/or Zambia) be better off if the Sport for Hope Centres had not been constructed? Why or why not?

5. Based on this case, what conclusions (if any) can be drawn regarding the general benefits and limitations of international sport-related development projects carried out in the wake of natural or man-made disasters?

6. What strategies could sport organizations like the IOC use to better manage public perceptions and interpretations of projects like the Sport for Hope program?

REFERENCES

Abrahamson, A. (2014, September 22). Sports and politics do mix. Retrieved from http://www.3wiresports.com/2014/09/24/sports-politics-mix/

Associated Press. (2010, October 25). IOC plans Olympics center, 'lasting legacy' for Haiti. *USA Today*. [Website]. Retrieved from http://usatoday30.usatoday.com/sports/olympics/2010-10-25-ioc-plans-olympic-center-for-haiti_N.htm

Beacom, A. (2012). *International diplomacy and the Olympic movement: The new mediators*. Basingstoke, UK: Palgrave Macmillan.

Bell, B. (2013). *Fault lines: Views across Haiti's divide*. Ithaca, NY: Cornell University Press.

Brattberg, E., & Sundelius, B. (2011). Mobilizing for international disaster relief: Comparing U.S. and EU approaches to the 2010 Haiti earthquake. *Journal of Homeland Security and Emergency Management, 8,* 1-22.

Butler, N. (2014a, July 15). Sport for Hope Centre in Haiti opened by IOC president in latest example of sport boosting wider development. Retrieved from Inside the Games. [Website].

http://www.insidethegames.biz/articles/1021320/sport-for-hope-centre-in-haiti-opened-by-ioc-president-in-latest-example-of-sport-boosting-wider-development

Butler, N. (2014b, August 27). Zambian 100m victory highlights success of Sport for Hope Centre in Lusaka. Inside the Games. [Website]. Retrieved from http://www.insidethegames.biz/articles/1022178/zambian-100m-victory-highlights-success-of-sport-for-hope-centre-in-lusaka

Charles, J. (2015, January 11). Tens of thousands still living in tents 5 years after Haiti earthquake. *Miami Herald.* Retrieved from http://www.miamiherald.com/news/nation-world/world/americas/haiti/article6005817.html

Charles, J., Clark, L., & Robes, F. (2010, January 15). Haiti's desperation rises as swell of bodies grows. *Philadelphia Inquirer.* Retrieved from http://articles.philly.com/2010-01-15/news/24956170_1_bodies-morgue-rescue-workers

CSA Group. (2012, February 14). Haiti's Sports for Hope Olympic center groundbreaking. CSA Group. [Website]. Retrieved from http://www.csagroup.com/news_piece.php?nid=38

Dantò, E. (2015, January 11). Haiti "reconstruction": Land grabbing, privatization and occupation. *GlobalResearch: Centre for Research on Globalization.* Retrieved from http://www.globalresearch.ca/haiti-reconstruction-anti-imperialist-leaders-collaborating-with-the-u-s-empire-in-land-grabbing-privatization-and-occupation/5378164

Dayan, J. (1995). *Haiti, history, and the gods.* Berkeley, CA: University of California Press.

General Electric. (2014, August). GE LED lighting brightens "Sports for Hope" Centre in Haiti. Retrieved from http://www.gelighting.com/LightingWeb/la_en/south/projects/sports-for-hope-centre-haiti.jsp

Giardina, M. D., & Cole, C. L. (2012). Race, class, and politics in post-Katrina America. In D. L. Andrews & M. L. Silk (Eds.), *Sport and neoliberalism: Politics, consumption, and culture* (pp. 57-74). Philadelphia, PA: Temple University Press.

Guttmann, A. (1984). *The games must go on: Avery Brundage and the Olympic movement.* New York, NY: Columbia University Press.

Hancock, G. (1989). *Lords of poverty: The power, prestige, and corruption of the international aid business.* New York, NY: The Atlantic Monthly Press.

International Association of Athletics Federations. (2014, July 16). Sport for Hope Centre opens in Haiti. Retrieved from http://www.iaaf.org/news/iaaf-news/sport-for-hope-centre-haiti-ioc-mondo

International Monetary Fund. (2015). World economic outlook database. [Website database]. Retrieved from http://www.imf.org/external/pubs/ft/weo/2015/02/weodata/weoselgr.aspx

International Olympic Committee. (2010a). *Sports for Hope: Olympic Youth Development Centre – Lusaka, Zambia.* Lausanne, Switzerland. Retrieved from http://www.olympic.org/Documents/Commissions_PDFfiles/sports-for-hope-brochure.pdf

International Olympic Committee. (2010b). *IOC inaugurates first Olympic Youth Development Centre in Lusaka, Zambia.* Retrieved from http://www.olympic.org/news/ioc-inaugurates-first-olympic-youth-development-centre-in-lusaka-zambia/88825

International Olympic Committee. (2012). *After Lusaka, a second Olympic centre is to be created—in Haiti.* Retrieved from http://www.olympic.org/news/after-lusaka-a-secondolympic-centre-is-to-be-created-in-haiti/

International Olympic Committee. (2014a). *IOC and UN Secretariat agree historic deal to work together to use sport to build a better world.* Retrieved from http://www.olympic.org/news/ioc-and-un-secretariat-agree-historic-deal/230542

International Olympic Committee. (2014b). *Olympic Agenda 2020: 20+20 recommendations.* Lausanne, Switzerland. Retrieved from http://www.olympic.org/Documents/Olympic_Agenda_2020/Olympic_Agenda_2020-20-20_Recommendations-ENG.pdf

International Olympic Committee. (2015a). *Olympic Charter.* Lausanne, Switzerland. Retrieved from http://www.olympic.org/Documents/olympic_charter_en.pdf

International Olympic Committee. (2015b, July 15). Sport for Hope Centre in Haiti celebrates first anniversary. Retrieved from http://www.olympic.org/news/sport-for-hope-centre-in-haiti-celebrates-first-anniversary/246553

Johnston, J. (2015a, January 21). Is USAID helping Haiti to recover, or US contractors to make millions? *The Nation.* Retrieved from http://www.thenation.com/article/usaid-helping-haiti-recover-or-us-contractors-make-millions/

Johnston, J. (2015b, March 5). How the US plan to build houses for displaced Haitians became an epic boondoggle. *Vice.* Retrieved from https://news.vice.com/article/how-the-us-plan-to-build-houses-for-displaced-haitians-became-an-epic-boondoggle

Kelman, I. (2012). *Disaster diplomacy: How disasters affect peace and conflict.* New York, NY: Routledge.

Kilgore, A. (2015, July 29). Want to host the Olympics? Most western cities would rather not. *Washington Post.* Retrieved from https://www.washingtonpost.com/sports/olympics/for-citizens-in-many-locales-hosting-games-no-longer-has-same-ring-to-it/2015/07/29/10ac4c12-355a-11e5-94ce-834ad8f5c50e_story.html

Klein, N. (2007). *The shock doctrine: The rise of disaster capitalism.* New York, NY: Metropolitan Books.

Krause, M. (2014). *The good project: Humanitarian relief NGOs and the fragmentation of reason.* Chicago, IL: University of Chicago Press.

Loewenstein, A. (2015). *Disaster capitalism: Making a killing out of catastrophe.* Brooklyn, NY: Verso Books.

Middleton, N., & O'Keefe, P. (1998). *Disaster and development: The politics of humanitarian aid.* London, UK: Pluto Press.

Nikolova, E., & Marinov, N. (2015, April 22). How disaster relief can increase corruption. *Washington Post.* Retrieved from https://www.washingtonpost.com/blogs/monkey-cage/wp/2015/04/22/how-disaster-relief-can-increase-corruption/

Oxfam International. (2011). *From relief to recovery: Supporting good governance in post-earthquake Haiti.* Oxford, UK: Martin Hartberg, Aurelie Proust, & Michael Bailey.

Robles, F. (2012, January 10). Questions arise about how Haiti earthquake donations have been spent. *Miami Herald.* Retrieved from http://www.miamiherald.com/news/local/community/article1939300.html

Simmons, S. (2014, May 15). Bermane Stiverne is Canada's mystery world boxing champ. *Toronto Sun.* Retrieved from http://www.torontosun.com/2014/05/15/bermane-stiverne-is-canadas-mystery-world-boxing-champ

Thomson, S. (2015, January 12). Haiti's healing far from finished 5 years after deadly earthquake. Retrieved from http://www.cbc.ca/m/touch/world/story/1.2897785

Times of Zambia. (2015, February 13). Zambia: Should SCZ, NOC merge? [Website]. Retrieved from http://allafrica.com/stories/201502150010.html

UN General Assembly, 69th Session. (2014, October 16). Resolution A/69/L.5, *Sport as a means to promote education, health, development and peace.* Retrieved from http://www.un.org/ga/search/view_doc.asp?symbol=A/69/l.5

United Nations. (2010). *Final report of the independent panel of experts on the cholera outbreak in Haiti.* New York, NY: Alejandro Cravioto, Claudio Lanata, Daniele S. Lantagne, & G. Balakrish Nair.

United Nations Office for the Coordination of Humanitarian Affairs. (2015). *Financial tracking service: Tracking global humanitarian aid flows.* Retrieved from https://fts.unocha.org

United Nations Office on Sport for Development and Peace. (2012). *Zambia, the playing field for further UN-Olympic cooperation.* Retrieved from http://www.un.org/wcm/content/site/sport/home/newsandevents/news/template/news_item.jsp?cid=32705

Weisbrot, M. (2011, April 22). Haiti and the international aid scam. *The Guardian.* Retrieved from http://www.theguardian.com/commentisfree/cifamerica/2011/apr/22/haiti-aid

Zambian Watchdog. (2013, June 19). OYDC in financial and other scandals. Retrieved from http://www.zambiawatchdog.com/oydc-in-financial-and-other-scandals/

Zimbalist, A. (2015). *Circus maximus: The economic gamble behind hosting the Olympics and the World Cup.* Washington, D.C.: Brookings Institution Press.

6

FROM "DIPLOMATIC DWARF" TO GULLIVER UNBOUND? BRAZIL AND THE USE OF SPORTS MEGA-EVENTS

CLAUDIO ROCHA · JONATHAN GRIX

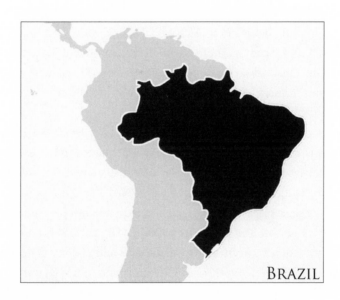

BRAZIL

On July 8th, 2014, Israel launched a massive military attack in the Gaza Strip, which has been ruled by Hamas, a Palestinian Islamic organization, since 2005, when Israel withdrew its army from this territory. Israel accused Hamas of starting the conflict by firing rockets from Gaza to Israel. After weeks of bombardment, 1,881 Palestinian and 67 Israeli citizens died (Yourish & Keller, 2014). International organizations accused both sides of many human rights violations and urged for a cease fire (Human Rights Watch, 2014).

Worldwide, most countries manifested support for Israel based on the fact that Hamas started the conflict (*National Post,* 2014). The United States, for example, supported its long-term allies, by sending $225 million in military aid to Israel (Everett, 2014). But what caused disquiet in the international media was the fact that Brazil's Foreign Ministry condemned the "escalation of violence," urged an end to the conflict, and added, "We strongly condemn the disproportionate use of force by Israel in the Gaza Strip" (Tavener, 2014, p.1). Israel did not like the statement and its Foreign Ministry spokesman suggested, "This is an unfortunate demonstration of why Brazil, an economic and cultural giant, remains a diplomatic dwarf" (Keinon, 2014, p. 7). Curiously, the international press did not consider this as the worst insult directed at Brazil (Taylor, 2014). The Israeli spokesman added, "This is not football. In football, when a game ends in a draw, you think it is proportional, but when it finishes 7-1, it's disproportionate. Sorry to say, but not so in real life and under international law" (Taylor, 2014).

The diplomat was referring to the humiliating defeat Brazil had suffered to Germany in one of the semi-finals of the home-hosted 2014 FIFA World Cup, in the very same month of that Gaza conflict. For many sport media persons, this was one of the worst and most embarrassing sporting defeats ever (McNulty, 2014). Clearly, in using a very bitter loss in sport, the Israeli spokesman meant to offend Brazil. But should Brazil take more offense on being called a diplomatic dwarf or a sporting contest loser? Even more intriguing is why the international media spread the second comment so intensely and considered it even more offensive than the first one.

Following a recent trend among developing countries, Brazil bid and won the rights to host the 2014 FIFA World Cup and the 2016 Olympic Games, in Rio de Janeiro. The country has many and diverse political motivations to host such events. Certainly among these motivations, improving its diplomatic role in international affairs is a very important one. Historically, hosting sport mega-events has represented a unique opportunity to improve public diplomacy (Black & Van Der Westhuizen, 2004). The current hosting trend is the third wave of the connection between sports mega-events and diplomacy development. The first wave happened after World War II, when the Axis countries hosted three Olympic Games in a period of sixteen years (Rome 1960, Tokyo 1964, and Munich, 1972) in an attempt to send a message of recovery to the rest of the world (Black & Van Der Westhuizen, 2004). The second wave came in the 1960s through the 1990s, when postcolonial countries used both sport mega-events (Mexico City 1968 and Seoul 1988 Olympic Games) and international events (South Africa 1995 Rugby World Cup and Malaysia 1998 Commonwealth Games) to indicate industrial, economic, and social progress. The third wave started with the Beijing 2008 Olympic Games and passed through South Africa 2010 and Brazil 2014 FIFA World Cups, Sochi 2014 Winter Olympics, and the Rio de Janeiro 2016 Olympic Games. Considering that Russia and Qatar will host the 2018 and 2022 FIFA World Cups, respectively, this third wave continues.

This chapter offers an assessment of Brazil's political use of not one but two sports mega-events, and considers whether hosting the most prestigious and globally recognized and watched sporting events will see the country move beyond the "diplomatic dwarf" stereotype touched on above. The chapter unfolds as follows: first, we situate the debate on Brazil among the wider literature on sports mega-events and the renaissance of sport and diplomacy studies. We then discuss the diplomatic problems facing Brazil, before looking specifically at Brazil's double host status and what this may mean for the nation.

SPORTS MEGA-EVENTS AND DIPLOMATIC STUDIES

Much ink has been spilled discussing sports mega-events, including the legacies they are supposed to produce (Preuss, 2007), the leveraging strategies states adopt to get at such legacies (Chalip, 2006), the politics and the political use of these events (Grix, 2013), the economic benefits states can gain through hosting (Gratton, Shibli, & Coleman, 2006), and the impact of major sporting events on citizens and their attitudes towards sport and physical activity (Weed M., Coren, E., Fiore, J., Wellard, I., Mansfield, L., Chatziefstathiou, D., & Dowse, S. 2012). A differentiation in the literature is along the lines of type of states hosting (advanced capitalist versus emerging states) and among the events themselves, with the Olympics and the FIFA World Cup—both of which Brazil were charged with hosting—generally seen as sports megas of the first order and thus, globally the most prestigious and sought-after (on emerging states see Grix and Lee, 2013; for a categorization of sports mega-events see Black, 2008). Thus, the case of Brazil dealt with in this chapter is one of an emerging state taking on the double host status of the world's largest sporting spectacles.

It is fair to say that the academic literature on sport and politics in general is relatively thin on the ground; the literature on international relations (IR) and sport and diplomacy and sport, in particular, is even thinner. Recently, there has been an increase in IR and sport and diplomacy in sport, the latter drawing on Joseph Nye's concept of soft power (Brannagan & Giulianotti, 2014; Cornelissen, 2010; Manzenreiter, 2010; Nygård & Gates, 2013). Scholars have turned to Nye's concept as a lens through which to explain why states host sports mega-events in terms of their place in the international arena. What binds both emerging and advanced capitalist states when hosting sports megas is the attempt to leverage the occasion to (a) improve a tarnished image (e.g., Germany, South Africa etc.); (b) put their states on the international map (e.g., Qatar, South Korea); (c) signal to the world their growing economic, diplomatic, and/or political strength (e.g., China, Russia, etc.); and (d) to show the watching world that they, the hosts, can put on what is one of the most logically complex events that exists. Of course, these reasons are not mutually exclusive and many states seek to use the event to achieve all of the above. The Brazilian state does not have a tarnished image, as Germany had prior to 2006 and their hosting of the FIFA World Cup. While Brazil is already on the world stage, it seeks to step out of the shadow of its depiction as a "diplomatic dwarf." The double-host status of Brazil is designed to send a signal that Brazil has finally arrived and now punches its weight; finally, pulling off both events without any major hitches will send out a message that Brazil is ready to do business with the most advanced states in the world.

CURRENT DIPLOMATIC CHALLENGES OF BRAZIL

In 2015, Brazil ranks as the world's fifth-largest landmass, fifth-largest population, and seventh-largest economy. Brazil has been considered an emergent power since 2001, when a Goldman Sachs report coined the term BRIC (Brazil, Russia, India, and China) to refer to the group of growth markets that nowadays accounts for about 20% of global gross domestic product and is expected to overtake the U.S. economy by the next decade (Bodman, Wolfensohn, & Sweig, 2011; Malamud, 2011). Despite the recent reduction in the economic growth of these nations, the BRICs kept working together to turn the positive predictions into reality. In 2014, they agreed to start a $50 billion "BRICs Bank" to invest in developing nations projects, alongside a $100 billion pool of reserve (Kenny, 2014). Brazil has also been part of the so-called IBSA alliance along with India and South Africa since 2003. Basically, these three countries have been lobbying for reforms at the United Nations and looking for a stronger participation of developing countries (Flemes, 2009). The emergence of Brazil as a global actor has attracted the attention of the United States, the European Union, and the G-8, which have been calling Brazil a "strategic partner" in their diplomatic meetings.

The increased importance of Brazil in the international political scenario in the last decade has changed the country's diplomatic aspirations. The country has not hidden its major diplomatic aspiration: to have a permanent seat on the United Nations Security Council (UNSC). France, United Kingdom, and Russia have supported Brazil's intentions, while the United States and China remained uncommitted in their support (Brown, 2012). However, in 2011, an independent task force of the Council of Foreign Relations analyzed Brazil-U.S. relationships and recommended that U.S. policymakers should recognize Brazil as a global actor and support its bid for a permanent seat on the UNSC (Bodman et al., 2011). The basis for this recommendation is that the US has exercised unilateral influence in South America since the 1800s (Brown, 2012); therefore, that task force indicated that practical steps, like supporting Brazil on the UNSC, would signal a more mature relationship with the "new" Brazil (Bodman et al., 2011). This recommendation has not been implemented so far.

There are at least two recent decisions made by Brazilian diplomats that have created a sense of suspicion in U.S. authorities regarding supporting Brazil on the UNSC. First, in 2010, as a nonpermanent member of the Council, Brazil voted against implementing sanctions on Iran (and indirectly against the US). The Security Council was imposing additional sanctions on Iran because of its alleged "lack of compliance with previous resolutions on ensuring the peaceful nature of its nuclear program" (United Nations, 2010, p. 1). Brazil explained its vote in affirming that additional sanctions "would lead to the suffering of the Iranian people and play into the hands of those on all sides who did not want a peaceful resolution of the issue" (United Nations, 2010, p. 4). Second, in 2011, Brazil along with Germany, Russia, China, and India abstained from voting on tightened sanctions on Libya and stressed "the need for peaceful resolution of the conflict and warned against unintended consequences of armed intervention" (United Nations, 2011, p. 3). The conflict referred to was the Libyan civil war, which broke out in 2011.

According to Brown (2012), in both instances Brazil showed coherence with its diplomatic values of nonmilitary intervention as far as possible. Although Brazil's military budget exceeded all other South American nations combined (Malamud, 2011), the country has decided to rely heavily on soft power to conquer its international space. Malamud (2011) noted that Brazil's market size, enormous exports, and investment potential have been effective in international affairs. Recent events have reinforced Brazil's option to rely on soft power when planning diplomatic growth.

Cason and Power (2009) claimed that, since 1995, the changes in Brazilian foreign policies have been rooted in international, national, or individual levels (as proposed by Waltz, 1959). The end of the cold war (international level), the resurgence of democracy (national level), and the election of two presidents (individual level) who focused on the changing Brazilian role in the international arena have changed Brazil's foreign policy. Cason and Power added that the "presidentialization" of Brazilian international affairs—mainly conducted by the two last presidents, Fernando Henrique Cardoso (1995-2002) and Luiz Inacio Lula da Silva (2003-2010)—had positive impacts on Brazil's profile on the world stage. Both presidents worked to strengthen the "Mercosul"—the free trade agreement between Brazil, Argentina, Uruguay, Paraguay, and Venezuela. During his term, President Lula constantly expressed a deep desire to see a stronger South America and believed that Brazil's leadership would be fundamental to creating a better continent (Cason & Power, 2009).

Not by chance, during Lula's term, Brazil was chosen to host the 2014 FIFA World Cup and the 2016 Olympic Games (in Rio de Janeiro). Some authors argue that the involvement of the president in the Olympic bid was fundamental in convincing the IOC to grant, for the first time ever, the Olympic Games to a South American country (Carey, Mason, & Misener, 2011). The fact that Brazil was chosen as the host of the 2014 World Cup was not as important as the fact it was chosen as the host of the 2016 Olympics. In fact, other South American countries (including Brazil itself) have hosted previous editions of the FIFA World Cup (e.g., Uruguay, Chile, and Argentina).

Since 2007, Brazil has used international sports events as part of its strategy to expand its soft power, diplomacy, and international relevance. Only in the last ten years, the country hosted the 2007 Pan-American Games, the 2011 Military World Games, the 2013 Confederations Cup, the 2014 FIFA World Cup, and the 2016 Rio Olympic Games. While the three former events have been called second-order sport events (Black & Van Der Westhuizen, 2004), they can be understood as a necessary precursor to hosting first-order events, the latter two are definitely the most important global sporting events in the world. Consequently, these events have brought unprecedented media attention to the host country. In the next section, we discuss how Brazil can use these sports mega-events to expand its soft power and grow in diplomatic stature.

BRAZIL, SPORT MEGA-EVENTS, AND DIPLOMACY

Brazil has tried to use the promotional effects of the 2014 World Cup and the 2016 Olympic Games to expand its soft power and diplomatic status. The literature supports the idea of positive relationships between hosting sport mega-events and increasing soft power (Finlay & Xin, 2010; Grix, Brannagan, & Houlihan, 2015). As suggested by Grix et al. (2015), successfully hosting sport mega-events "is increasingly acknowledged to be a highly visible and potential positive signal to other countries, acting as a valuable asset in accelerating their entry to, and acceptance within, the world's mature economies" (p. 470). Soft power is directly related to public diplomacy, since both involve the ability of having influence over others via attraction instead of coercion (Nye, 2008). Therefore, in expanding its soft power by hosting sport mega-events, Brazil is actually looking to improve its public diplomacy. Cornelissen (2010) asserted that Olympic Games and World Cups have been used by developing countries "to showcase economic achievements, to signal diplomatic stature or to project, in the absence of other forms of international influence, soft power" (p. 3008).

However, Grix et al. (2015) proposed that Brazil is not a typical case of an emerging nation using the association with sport mega-events to increase soft power and improve public diplomacy. They argued that Brazil is different because it is already "at the forefront of the emerging powers discourse" (p. 474) and it is using the mega-events to shift from a regional leader to a global leader. In agreement with this statement, Malamud (2011) reported that Brazil's role as an emergent global player has been confirmed by some invitations from important international institutions. For example, in 2005, the G-8 formally invited five developing countries (Brazil, China, India, Mexico, and South Africa), in the so-called G-8+5, to join the group talks in the summit hosted in Gleneagles, Scotland. Two years later, the European Union invited Brazil for a strategic partnership, leaving other South American countries out. Naturally, Brazil's prominence has not resounded well among other South American nations, which have developed strategies to slow that rising path (Malamud, 2011). For instance, although a regional commercial partner, Argentina has not supported Brazil's aspirations to become a permanent member on the United Nations Security Council. According to Malamud, Brazil has found that global diplomatic ambition can prompt regional resentment, creating what he called "the mounting mismatch between the regional and global recognition of Brazilian status" (Malamud, 2011, p. 19).

From a diplomatic point of view, probably the most effective way to act would be to forget the regional leadership and focus on the global context (Cason & Power, 2009; Malamud, 2011). However, as mentioned previously, mainly during Lula's term, leading South America was almost an obsession. In this regard, hosting the Olympic Games has a special meaning. Since the bid campaign, Lula has proposed that the 2016 Olympics should be not only the Rio and Brazil Olympic Games, but the *South America* Games. The former president asserted, "It is time to make the Olympics democratic, developing countries have the right to host the Games.... South America has the right to hold the Games" (Bugge, 2009). Lula knew that no other country in South America would have the infrastructure and financial resources to compete for the Games. Therefore, he used the special economic moment of the country to bid for the Games and consolidate himself as a regional leader. Interestingly, Brazil did not use the 2014 FIFA World Cup in the same way, simply because it would not work with the World Cup. First, the World Cup has been previously hosted by other South American countries. Second, soccer is the preferred sport in the majority of the South American countries, which already have at least the initial infrastructure to host it. Finally, Brazilian leaders know that the World Cup will eventually be hosted by other South American countries, which is unlikely to happen with the Olympic Games, at least in the short term.

However, hosting the Olympic Games is not a guarantee of growing diplomatic power. Other emerging states have tried to use sport mega-events to attain this aim, but they have run into some trouble. For example, investigating the recent experiences of Russia (Sochi 2014) and China (Beijing 2008) with the Olympic Games, scholars highlighted controversial policies regarding human rights and the treatment of minorities that have hindered these countries' intentions to use the Olympics to accomplish diplomatic objectives (Arnold & Foxall, 2014; Manzenreiter, 2010). The negative aspect of hosting major games has been termed both a double-edged sword and soft disempowerment (Grix & Houlian, 2014; Brannagan, 2014). Both terms point to an effect opposite that states set out to achieve through hosting: rather than enhancing their global status, the media attention brought to bear on hosts magnifies negative aspects of a state's politics, culture, or human rights record. Qatar is a case in point: the initial jubilation on winning the hosting rights for the 2022 FIFA World Cup gave way, quickly, to full-scale investigative journalism into Qatar's treatment of their foreign workforce, frantically building sporting infrastructure from scratch.

Additionally, according to Manzenreiter (2010), hosting the 2008 Olympic Games did not change the antiquated and oppressive designs adopted by China to deal with Taiwan and Tibet. Therefore, considering that during the 2008 Olympics, the eyes of the world were on China, even those people who had not previously known about its insistence on state sovereignty and violations of human rights became aware of such problems. Apparently, such exposition made diplomatic relationships between China and Western countries more complicated (Manzenreiter, 2010). Similarly, the 2014 Sochi Winter Olympics brought more decline than improvement for Russia in terms of diplomatic relationships. The controversial law that prohibited "propaganda of nontraditional sexual relations" exposed Russia's intolerance toward the LGBT community became the most-commented-on human right violation in the international press in 2014 (Arnold & Foxall, 2014). In addition to the state-sponsored homophobia, during the preparation for Sochi 2014, Russia faced other problems (such as journalism censure and the arrest of Greenpeace activists), which damaged its project to send a positive image of the country abroad in association with the Olympics (Simons, 2014). Taken together, Russia's use of sports mega-events, like Brazil's, does not fit the usual explanation of simply trying to showcase their nation and increase soft power via sporting spectacles. Russia's use of sports megas is less about sport diplomacy and much more part of a special governance strategy (Grix and Kramavera, 2015; see also "Putin and the 2014 Winter Olympics: Russia's Authoritarian Sports Diplomacy" in this book).

DOUBLE-EDGED SWORD FOR BRAZIL?

On the one hand, Brazil has seemingly avoided controversies related to violations of human and minority rights, but on the other hand, the country has suffered historically from a culture of corruption. More recently, two impressive cases of corruption emerged, affecting politicians of all levels, including two former presidents of the republic. The first case of corruption affected the credibility of the then-president Luiz Inacio Lula da Silva, when in 2005, a vote-buying scheme named "mensalao" (big money stipend) was discovered inside the national congress (*The Economist,* 2013). After years of prosecution, the second most powerful man of Brazil at that time and the right-hand man of Lula, Jose Dirceu, went to jail in 2013, sending a positive message domestically and internationally about Brazil's serious intentions to combat corruption (*The Economist,* 2013). Unfortunately, another corruption scheme has erupted in Brazil in 2015. Since then, a bribery scheme involving Petrobras, the state oil company, has placed a lot of supporters of the former president Ms. Dilma Rousseff under investigation. Most of these supporters belong to the left Worker's Party, the party of former president Lula (Segal, 2015). Many politicians are still under investigation, but the apex of the case was reached in August 2016, when Ms. Roussef was impeached and removed from office.

Such cases of corruption have produced some popular manifestations against the government. For example, during the Confederations Cup in 2013, many protests and riots against corruption happened in different places in the country, mainly in the host cities of this event (Watts, 2014; Zirin, 2013). In October 2015, ten months before the 2016 Olympic Games, more protests against corruption in the federal government erupted in Brazilian streets (Biller & Colitt, 2015). Most of the protesters involved in such resistance have requested the impeachment of the President Dilma Rousseff, mainly because of her alleged involvement in the bribery scheme of Petrobras. Because sport mega-events have brought Brazil into the international spotlight, such manifestations and their consequences may signal that Brazil is finally fighting corruption seriously. In this sense, sport mega-events can help Brazil to be better perceived by other nations as a serious international player, not only because it is able to host such events, but also and mainly because it is able and willing to battle corruption.

Spalding et al. (2014) affirmed that the 2014 World Cup and the 2016 Olympic Games have drawn, and will draw, "the world's attention to a nation's anti-corruption efforts as few events ever could" (p. 2). These authors added that "Brazil has become a kind of vortex for the global anti-corruption movement," because "its popular protests and governmental response in the form of specific legal reforms" (p. 3). In fact, the government response to the public outcry seems to be somehow linked to the fact that Brazil is in the international spotlight because of the sport mega-events. That is, the Brazilian government has felt the pressure of so much international exposure and started to support, at least symbolically, measures against corruption. In practice, as shown above, the federal government is highly involved in corruption scandals (Segal, 2015). However, as noted by the international press, the Brazilian Federal Supreme Court has been more efficient than ever in trying to condemn politicians, lobbyists, and businessmen for corruption (*The Economist,* 2013). Meanwhile, scholars have mentioned that Brazil's democratic institutions, independent judiciary, and free press have made the country more likely to improve its diplomacy via battling corruption when hosting the events; especially if someone compares it to previous hosts, such as Russia/Sochi 2014 and China/Beijing 2008 (Spalding et al., 2014).

In this sense, the current status of Brazilian institutions in association with the international attention received by the country has helped Brazil to promote itself as a less corrupt nation. However, the association with FIFA and the IOC can bring a reverse effect. Both institutions have been frequently involved with corruption in the remote and recent past (Abrahamson, 1999; Zirin, 2014). For instance, Joseph "Sepp" Blatter, FIFA president for the last 17 years, has recently resigned due to intense pressure from investigations by the FBI and Swiss prosecutors that have led to 18 senior soccer executives being charged on accusations of money laundering and tax evasion (Gibson, 2015). The closer a country is associated with these organizations, the more they are likely to be suspected of involvement in corruption (Spalding et al., 2014). For example, Germany was recently accused of buying the right to host the 2006 World Cup (Smith, 2015). According to German newspaper *Der Spiegel,* the bid committee bribed four Asian representatives with about US $11 million to vote for Germany's candidature (Smith, 2015). Similarly, Qatar has been constantly accused of buying votes to be chosen as the host of the 2022 FIFA World Cup (Brannagan & Giulianotti, 2014). Likewise, the 2014 Winter Olympic Games in Sochi has brought a lot of corruption accusations over Russia. As noted by Arnold and Foxall (2014), "the astronomical cost of the Sochi 2014 Olympic Games [US $51 billion] is an indictment of the pervasive corruption in the Russian system" (p. 6). Therefore, the challenge of Brazil is to use the international media interest before, during, and after the World Cup and the Olympics to showcase its fight against corruption, while avoiding FIFA and IOC corruption scandals.

Considering that the 2014 World Cup has already passed, in terms of sport policies, Brazilian authorities have focused on creating an environment in the country that helps national athletes to perform the best they can during the 2016 Olympic Games. They believe that an outstanding performance of the national athletes might improve the country's image internationally. Rhamey and Early (2013) support this belief when they reported that good performances in the Olympic Games (i.e., winning a lot of medals) would build a positive image and enhance the international prestige of any nation. Additionally, these authors found that both surpassing the expectations in Olympic performance (winning medals) and hosting the event would produce the greatest gains in terms of improving diplomatic contacts with other nations.

The decision to host sport mega-events is an attempt to break a virtual circle in elite sport in Brazil—to date, low investments have produced low performances. Brazil has had a very flat performance in terms of medals won in the Olympics. For example, in the last two Games—2012 London and 2008 Beijing—Brazil won 17 and 15 medals, finishing in the 23rd and 22nd position, respectively. For the 2016 Games, Brazilian sport authorities have established the goal of finishing among the top 10 (ESPN, 2015). In order to achieve this aim, they know much more investment needs to be put into sport. In hosting the 2016 Games, the local sport authorities have seen an opportunity to increase investments in both sporting infrastructure and the preparation of elite athletes. Rocha (2015) described four different federal programs, which have been supporting the preparation of Team Brazil for the 2016 Olympics. About R$1 billion will be invested in athletes' preparation and physical structures and equipment between 2013 and 2016 (Brasil, 2014)—two thirds of this money has come from federal funds and one third from sponsorships of public enterprises to support the preparation of the national teams. For example, the national bank—"Banco do Brasil"—has sponsored the Brazilian teams in volleyball, beach volleyball, sailing, and modern pentathlon. Other public organizations have supported other sports in Brazil, as part of the preparation for the 2016 Olympic Games.

Such investments in elite sport and (the expected) outstanding performance in the 2016 Olympic Games can bring some benefits to Brazil in diplomatic terms (Rhamey & Early, 2013). However, internal policies related to human and social rights are considered much more important to measure the diplomatic stature of a country than winning medals or hosting events. In this sense, Brazil's strategy to focus heavily on elite sport, while relegating education and social sport to the status of a poor cousin may be a mistake, from a diplomatic point of view. The World Cup and the Olympic Games should be used to showcase a new Brazil, where sport is an important tool not only to produce better elite athletes, but also—and mainly—to promote well-being, social rights, gender equity, and diversity. Unfortunately, the social and educational sport programs in the country have received fewer resources than the elite sport programs (Rocha, 2015). Only China, among the so-called emerging states, has been able to put on a spectacular Olympic event and top the Olympic medal table. Success in elite sport requires lots of resources over an extended period of time; it also requires a coordinated sports system with high quality school and community sport. Brazil is a long way from fulfilling these requirements.

FINAL REMARKS

Brazil has struggled to be perceived as a higher-stature actor in international affairs. The country's most important diplomatic aspiration remains to have a permanent seat on the United Nations Security Council. So far Brazil has not been successful in its attempts to accomplish this and a number of other aims related to international affairs. Currently, Brazil has attempted to use the 2014 World Cup and will use the 2016 Olympic Games to expand its soft power and diplomatic status. Hosting sports megas has been acknowledged as an important strategy to send messages of economic maturity and diplomatic importance to other international states (Grix et al., 2015).

Comparing Brazil to other developing nations that have recently used similar strategies, we note that the nation has had relative success in avoiding overt negative publicity, mainly related to violations of human and minority rights (which were frequently linked to China and Russia during the 2008 Beijing Games and the 2014 Sochi Winter Games). However, as we have pointed out, the constant media scrutiny that accompanies the hosting of a global sporting spectacle can reveal to the world more than just positive aspects of a country. For example, the media focus on Brazil has exposed many cases of corruption (despite the fact that corruption is endemic in this country). Moreover, Brazil has not escaped criticisms related to environment deterioration. The literature has reported the impact of construction of Olympic facilities on environmentally protected areas of Rio de Janeiro city and a pervasive concern about real estate speculation (Gaffney, 2013). In this sense, hosting sports mega-events and receiving extensive media coverage can be a double-edged sword for Brazil. Dealing with negative coverage, while reinforcing the positive aspects of the country is a difficult mission, which needs to be quickly accomplished if it wants to use the sports mega-events as catalysts for its diplomatic growth.

Finally, we argue that successfully hosting the sport mega-events and handling media coverage in a positive way might not be sufficient to elevate the current diplomatic status of Brazil. These events have brought a lot of attention to competitive sport and much has been invested in this area. Consequently, given the limited resources overall, little has been invested in educational and social sport programs. When the party is over, the medals are counted, and the Olympic caravan moves on, Brazil might not accrue all possible diplomatic benefits from hosting sports mega-events because of its focus on investing large amounts of money in sports stadia and promoting elite sport. We would suggest a better investment balance between elite sport, on the one hand, and social and educational sport programs, on the other. This is based on the fact that internal policies related to human and social rights are considered much more important to measure the diplomatic stature of a country than winning medals or hosting events.

DISCUSSION QUESTIONS

1. What is your perception about Brazil's current diplomatic status?
2. Do you believe that the 2014 World Cup and the 2016 Olympic Games had the same types of impact on the country, internally and internationally?
3. Thinking about legacies in general, do you think that hosting the two largest sport events in such a short period was strategically beneficial for Brazil? Why?
4. Do you think that hosting the 2014 World Cup and the 2016 Olympic Games has helped Brazil to improve its diplomatic status? Why?
5. Point out three benefits Brazil has reaped from hosting the 2016 Olympic Games.
6. Point out three criticisms Brazil has suffered for having hosted the 2016 Olympic Games.
7. Based on Brazil's experience, should other Latin American countries bid for the Olympic Games?

REFERENCES

Abrahamson, A. (1999). Australian paid IOC members in Sydney bid. *LA Times*. Retrieved from http://articles.latimes.com/1999/jan/23/news/mn-875

Arnold, R., & Foxall, A. (2014). Lord of the (Five) Rings. Issues at the 2014 Sochi Olympic Games. *Problems of Post-Communism, 61*, 3–12. Retrieved from http://doi.org/10.2753/PPC1075-8216610100

Biller, D., & Colitt, R. (2015). More than a million hit Brazil streets to protest Rousseff. *Bloomberg Business*. Retrieved from http://www.bloomberg.com/news/articles/2015-03-15/tens-of-thousands-march-in-brazil-streets-to-protest-rousseff

Black, D. (2008). Dreaming big: The pursuit of "second order games as a strategic response to globalization." *Sport in Society, 11*(4), 467–480.

Black, D., & Van Der Westhuizen, J. (2004). The allure of global games for 'semi-peripheral' polities and spaces: a research agenda. *Third World Quarterly, 25*, 1195–1214.

Bodman, S. W., Wolfensohn, J. D., & Sweig, J. E. (2011). *Global Brazil and US-Brazil relations. Independent task force report no. 66*. New York , NY: Council on Foreign Relations.

Brannagan, P. M., & Giulianotti, R. (2014). Soft power and soft disempowerment: Qatar, global sport and football's 2022 World Cup finals. *Leisure Studies,* (ahead-of-print), 1–17. Retrieved from http://doi.org/10.1080/02614367.2014.964291

Brasil. (2014). Website of "Ministério do Esporte do Brasil." Retrieved January 2, 2014, from http://www.esporte.gov.br/

Brown, L. T. (2012). *Restoring the "unwritten alliance" in Brazil-United States relations*. [Monograph]. Retrieved from http://www.dtic.mil/docs/citations/ADA560773

Bugge, A. (2009). South America deserves first Games in 2016, says Lula. *Reuters*. Retrieved from http://in.reuters.com/article/2009/04/03/idINIndia-38872620090403

Carey, M., Mason, D. S., & Misener, L. (2011). Social responsibility and the competitive bid process for major sporting events. *Journal of Sport & Social Issues, 35*, 246–263.

Cason, J. W., & Power, T. J. (2009). Presidentialization, pluralization, and the rollback of Itamaraty: Explaining change in Brazilian foreign policy making in the Cardoso-Lula era. *International Political Science Review, 30*, 117–140.

Chalip, L. (2006). Towards social leverage of sport events. *Journal of Sport & Tourism, 11*, 109–127.

Cornelissen, S. (2010). The geopolitics of global aspiration: Sport mega-events and emerging powers. *International Journal of the History of Sport, 27*, 3008–3025. Retrieved from <Go to ISI>://WOS:000290396200018

Economist, The. (2013). Political corruption in Brazil. Jail at last. *The Economist*. Retrieved from http://www.economist.com/news/americas/21590560-landmark-justice-jailed-last

ESPN. (2015). Por Top 10 em 2016, COB foca individuais e quer podio em 13 esportes. *ESPN Brasil*. Retrieved from http://espn.uol.com.br/noticia/494795_por-top-10-em-2016-cob-foca-individuais-e-quer-podio-em-13-esportes

Everett, B. (2014). Congress backs aid to Israel. *Politico*. Retrieved from http://www.politico.com/story/2014/08/senate-approves-israel-aid-109642.html

Finlay, C. J., & Xin, X. (2010). Public diplomacy games: A comparative study of American and Japanese responses to the interplay of nationalism, ideology and Chinese soft power strategies around the 2008 Beijing Olympics. *Sport in Society, 13*, 876–900.

Flemes, D. (2009). India-Brazil-South Africa (IBSA) in the New global order interests, strategies and values of the emerging coalition. *International Studies, 46*, 401–421.

Gaffney, C. (2013). Between discourse and reality: The unsustainability of mega-event planning. *Sustainability, 5*, 3926–3940.

Gibson, O. (2015). Sepp Blatter to resign as FIFA president after 17 years in role. *The Guardian*. Retrieved from http://www.theguardian.com/football/2015/jun/02 sepp-blatter-fifa-president-resigns

Gratton, C., Shibli, S., & Coleman, R. (2006). The economic impact of major sports events: A review of ten events in the UK. *The Sociological Review, 54*(S2), 41–58.

Grix, J. (2013). Sport politics and the Olympics. *Political Studies Review, 11*, 15–25.

Grix, J., Brannagan, P. M., & Houlihan, B. (2015). Interrogating states' soft power strategies: A case study of sports mega-events in Brazil and the UK. *Global Society, 29*, 463–479. Retrieved from http://doi.org/10.1080/13600826.2015.1047743

Grix, J., & Houlihan, B. (2014). Sports mega events as part of a nation's soft power strategy: The cases of Germany (2006) and the UK (2012). *The British Journal of Politics & International Relations, 16*(4), 572–596.

Grix, J., & Kramareva, N. (2015). The Sochi Winter Olympics and Russia's unique soft power strategy. *Sport in Society, 18*, 1–15.

Grix, J., & Lee, D. (2013). Soft power, sports mega-events and emerging states: The lure of the politics of attraction. *Global Society, 27*(4), 521–536.

Human Rights Watch. (2014). Palestine/Israel: Indiscriminate Palestinian rocket attacks. *Human Rights Watch News*. Retrieved from http://www.hrw.org/news/2014/07/09/palestineisrael-indiscriminate-palestinian-rocket-attacks

Keinon, H. (2014). Israel slams "diplomatic dwarf" Brazil for recalling envoy to protest Gaza operation. *The Jerusalem Post*. Retrieved from http://www.jpost.com/Operation-Protective-Edge/Brazil-recalls-ambassador-for-consultations-in-protest-of-IDF-Gaza-operation-368715

Kenny, C. (2014). The World's fastest-growing economies won't be scary unless they slow down. *Bloomberg Business*. Retrieved from http://www.bloomberg.com/bw/articles/2014-07-21/brics-summit-a-show-of-economic-might-is-nothing-to-fear

Malamud, A. (2011). A leader without followers? The growing divergence between the regional and global performance of Brazilian foreign policy. *Latin American Politics and Society, 53*(3), 1–24.

Manzenreiter, W. (2010). The Beijing games in the Western imagination of China: The weak power of soft power. *Journal of Sport & Social Issues, 34*, 29–48. http://doi.org/10.1177/0193723509358968

McNulty, P. (2014). Brazil's World Cup dreams ended in humiliating and brutal fashion as Germany inflicted their heaviest defeat in the first semi-final in Belo Horizonte. *BBC News*. Retrieved from www.bbc.com/sport/football/28102403

National Post. (2014). Stephen Harper accuses Hamas of using human shields, urges world leaders to side with Israel. *Canadian Press*. Retrieved from http://news.nationalpost.com/2014/07/13/stephen-harper-accuses-hamas-of-using-human-shields-urges-world-leaders-to-side-with-israel/

Nye, J. S. (2008). Public diplomacy and soft power. *The Annals of the American Academy of Political and Social Science, 616*, 94–109.

Nygård, H. M., & Gates, S. (2013). Soft power at home and abroad: Sport diplomacy, politics and peace-building. *International Area Studies Review, 16*, 235–243. Retrieved from http://doi.org/10.1177/2233865913502971

Preuss, H. (2007). The conceptualisation and measurement of mega sport event legacies. *Journal of Sport & Tourism, 12*(3), 207–227.

Rhamey, J. P., & Early, B. R. (2013). Going for the gold: Status-seeking behavior and Olympic performance. *International Area Studies Review, 16*, 244–261. Retrieved from http://doi.org/10.1177/2233865913499563

Rocha, C. M. (2015). Pubic sector and sport development in Brazil. In G. Bravo & R. L. Damico (Eds.), *Sport Policy and Management in Latin America*. Oxfordshire, UK: Routledge.

Segal, D. (2015). Petrobras oil scandal leaves Brazilians lamenting a lost dream. *The New York Times*. Retrieved from www.nytimes.com/2015/08/09/business/international/effects-of-petrobras-scandal-leave-brazilians-lamenting-a-lost-dream.html?_r=0

Simons, G. (2014). Russian public diplomacy in the 21st century: Structure, means and message. *Public Relations Review, 40*, 440–449. Retrieved from http://doi.org/http://dx.doi.org/10.1016/j.pubrev.2014.03.002

Smith, G. (2015). Did Germany bribe to win hosting rights to FIFA's 2006 World Cup? *Fortune.* Retrieved from http://fortune.com/2015/10/16/germany-fifa-2006-world-cup-bribe/

Spalding, A., Barr, P., Flores, A., Freiman, S., Gavin, K., Klink, T., ... Orden, R. Van. (2014). From the 2014 World Cup to the 2016 Olympics: Brazil's role in the global anti-corruption movement. *Southwestern Journal of International Law, 21,* 71–91.

Tavener, B. (2014). Though not a "diplomatic dwarf," Brazil lacks clout. *Aljazeera America.* Retrieved from http://america.aljazeera.com/opinions/2014/7/brazil-israel-dilmarousseffdiplomacygazais-rael.html

Taylor, A. (2014). Israel calls Brazil a "diplomatic dwarf"—and then brings up World Cup humiliation. *The Washington Post.* Retrieved from http://www.washingtonpost.com/blogs/worldviews/wp/2014/07/25/israel-brings-up-brazils-world-cup-humiliation-and-calls-the-country-a-diplomatic-dwarf/

United Nations. (2010). *Security Council Imposes Additional Sanctions on Iran, Voting 12 in Favour to 2 Against, with 1 Abstention.* Retrieved from http://www.un.org/press/en/2010/sc9948.doc.htm

United Nations. (2011). *Security council approves "no-fly zone" over Libya, authorizing "all necessary measures" to protect civilians, by vote of 10 in favour with 5 abstentions.* Retrieved from http://www.un.org/press/en/2011/sc10200.doc.htm

Waltz, K. N. (1959). *Man, the state and war: A theoretical analysis.* New York, NY: Columbia University Press.

Watts, J. (2014). Anti-world cup protests across Brazil. *The Guardian.* Retrieved from http://www.theguardian.com/world/2014/may/16/anti-world-cup-protests-across-brazil

Weed, M., Coren, E., Fiore, J., Wellard, I., Mansfield, L., Chatziefstathiou, D., & Dowse, S. (2012). Developing a physical activity legacy from the London 2012 Olympic and Paralympic Games: A policy-led systematic review. *Perspectives in Public Health, 132*(2), 75–80.

Yourish, K., & Keller, J. (2014). The toll in Gaza and Israel, day by day. *New York Times.* Retrieved from http://www.nytimes.com/interactive/2014/07/15/world/middleeast/toll-israel-gaza-conflict.html

Zirin, D. (2013). Brazil: Yes, blame the damn world cup. *The Nation.* Retrieved from http://www.thenation.com/blog/174947/brazil-yes-blame-damn-world-cup

Zirin, D. (2014). Throw FIFA out of the game. *New York Times.* Retrieved from http://www.nytimes.com/2014/06/08/opinion/sunday/throw-fifa-out-of-the-game.html

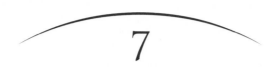

7

PUTIN AND THE 2014 SOCHI OLYMPICS: RUSSIA'S AUTHORITARIAN SPORTS DIPLOMACY

SUFIAN ZHEMUKHOV · ROBERT ORTTUNG

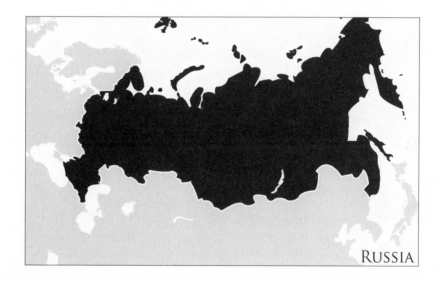

RUSSIA

INTRODUCTION

Russian President Vladimir Putin, a judo enthusiast and avid outdoorsman, frequently uses sports as a way to achieve his foreign diplomacy objectives. In autocratic Russia, such foreign efforts are closely intertwined with domestic policy goals. This chapter will examine how the Kremlin has sought to use sports mega-events like the Olympics to advance its agenda both at home and abroad. This first section examines the symbolic importance of sport in Russia. Second, we trace the post-Soviet history of Russia's efforts to host important sporting events. The third section lays out Putin's personal interest in sports. Fourth, we examine the international challenges to Russia in the run up to the games. Next, we consider the terrorist and security challenges faced in Sochi. Sixth, we look at the human rights violations surrounding the games. Subsequently, we consider Russia's actions immediately after the Olympics concluded, particularly the invasion of Crimea. Finally, the conclusion explains how Putin saw sporting mega-events as useful in his efforts to demonstrate that Russia's rightful place amongst the world's greatest powers.

THE SYMBOLIC IMPORTANCE OF THE 2014 SOCHI OLYMPICS

Sport plays a special role in international politics, and the Olympics are the pinnacle of this contribution. The games "became occasions for competitive national self-assertion," as Eric J. Hobsbawm, the famous theorist of modern nationalism, has noted (1990, p. 143). However, in addition to the competition with other nations that Hobsbawm discussed, the new Russia also competes with the past sporting achievements of the Soviet Union and uses sport to strengthen current leaders in the Kremlin.

The Kremlin's use of sports is multidimensional, but symbolism is where they provide the greatest payoff. Most importantly, sports contributed to building a new Russian identity after the fall of the Soviet Union. The Soviet leaders had used the 1980 Moscow Olympics as a stage to demonstrate the superiority of the Soviet system and the effectiveness of their Communist ideology. Soviet ideology claimed as its goal creating a new social order in which people would become more advanced, mentally and physically; the accomplishments of Soviet sportsmen were supposed to demonstrate the preeminence of the Soviet way of life (Alt & Alt, 1964).

Following the collapse of the Soviet Union, the post-Soviet Russian elite failed to create a new, comprehensive ideology, and contemporary Russia does not enjoy the prominent role that the Soviet Union used to play internationally. Soon after the fall of the Soviet Union, the first Russian president, Boris Yeltsin, claimed, "Great Russia is rising from its knees" (Yeltsin, 1991). Under Yeltsin's successor, Vladimir Putin, this approach developed into a new Russian state ideology, a phenomenon referred to as "the resurrection drama" (Persson & Petersson, 2013). Putin expressed the Russian sorrow for the loss of the Soviet empire in his 2005 statement, "the collapse of the Soviet Union was a major geopolitical disaster of the century. As for the Russian nation, it became a genuine drama" (Putin, 2005).

Lacking the ability to restore the Soviet Empire as it was, the Kremlin has tried to simulate such a restoration in symbolic ways. Most prominently, Putin's Kremlin restored the Soviet anthem as the new Russian national anthem in 2000 (Constitutional Federal Law of 25 December 2000, "On the State Anthem of the Russian Federation"). Current leaders of the Russian Federation also attempt to capitalize on sports in order to demonstrate that Russia is once again a strong international player that must be reckoned with.

Sporting events have become one of the means by which Russian society is able to deal with nostalgia for lost Soviet power. Russian politicians broadly refer to the 1980 Moscow Olympics as a reminder of the legacies of a great country, and references to the success of the Soviet hockey team in 1972 enhance the nostalgic propaganda of past glories (Makarychev, 2013). "Olympic sport was a creation of the state," Soviet Sport Historian Robert Edelman argued, "and could be molded regardless of the evolving tastes of the public" (Edelman, 1993, p. 126).

Yet, even as Russia deals with its Soviet past, the competition with other countries remains important. Here the final medal count is the yardstick for success. Considerable criticism followed the 2012 London Summer Olympics, when the U.S. team took first place with 46 gold medals and Russia was fourth with about half that number—24. Accordingly, Russia's ability to win the most medals of any country during the Sochi Olympics was particularly satisfying for the Russian audience.

POST-SOVIET OLYMPIC PROJECTS

Russia made many attempts to win the right to host the Olympics after East European communism began to collapse in 1988, demonstrating that the Olympics play a special role in Russia's symbolic competition with the past. Russian leaders were ready to spend tens of billions of dollars and many years of preparation for another Olympics in order to repeat the glory symbolized by the 1980 Moscow Olympics. Former Soviet President Mikhail Gorbachev and first Russian President Boris Yeltsin had little realistic chance to win an Olympic bid given the economic crises that defined their time in office. For Putin, who benefited from steadily rising oil prices during his first two terms, however, it was important to present the 2014 Olympics as the world's reward to Russia's leader for his ability to turn the economy around. Russia prepared numerous applications to hold the Olympics after 1980, but only achieved success with the 2014 Winter Olympics in Sochi.

As Russia became increasingly authoritarian after Putin's rise in 2000, the organizers of the 2014 Winter Olympics tried to link the Sochi Games personally to Putin rather than to previous efforts to host the Olympics in Russia. The organizers of the 2014 Sochi Winter Olympics rarely mentioned Russia's previous attempts to host the Olympics after 1980, including a previous failed effort to win the Winter Olympics for Sochi. This is despite the fact that referring to previous applications, including failed ones, is usual practice for most Olympic bids. Such references help build a history of consistency in attempts to hold the Olympics and demonstrate through persistence that a country (or city) gradually moved toward earning the right to host a big international mega-event like the Olympics. One of the explanations for why the organizers of the 2014 Olympics ignored Russia's previous efforts for hosting the Winter Games was that those projects were not connected to Putin personally. Thus the Sochi bid and related state propaganda avoided mentioning that, in 1986, Putin's hometown, St. Petersburg (then Leningrad), applied to host the 1994 Winter Olympics, but the Soviet Government cancelled the application at the last minute (Kavokin

& Evstifeev, 2015). This fact would seem significant since it was Putin's hometown that applied to host the Olympics. However, the organizers of the 2014 Olympics apparently could not find any evidence of Putin's personal involvement in St. Petersburg's 1986 proposal. Putin did not start working in decision-making positions in Leningrad until 1990, and when his hometown applied to host the Olympics in 1988, Putin was stationed as a KGB officer in East Germany.

In 1989, one year after St. Petersburg failed to win its bid for the Olympics, the National Olympic Committee of the Soviet Union initiated a bid to host the 1998 Winter Olympics in Sochi, but the Soviet Government did not approve this idea and it died before gaining much steam. It is even more striking than in the St. Petersburg case is that the organizers of the 2014 Olympics avoided mentioning the fact that Sochi itself had considered applying to host the 1998 Winter Olympics. The fact that the Soviet sport authorities regarded Sochi as an appropriate place for holding the Winter Olympics would have been a good argument against Putin's critics who disparaged the idea of hosting the 2014 Olympics in Sochi and argued that hosting winter games in a subtropical town was a bad idea. The opponents of the 2014 Sochi games wrote, "Russia is a winter country. It's hard to find a place on the Russian map where there has not been snow and where winter sports are not developed. But Putin found such a spot and decided to hold the Winter Olympics there. It's the city of Sochi" (Nemtsov & Martynyuk, 2013, p. 4). Also, Putin's critics argued that holding the Olympics in Sochi was not financially viable. And again, Putin failed to refer to a 1989 interview with the USSR Minister of Sport, Vitaly Smirnov, that addressed those issues, arguing that the Sochi mountains "hold snow nine months during the year" and that building a winter resort in Sochi would be "super-profitable" (Lamtsov, 1989).

After the fall of the Soviet Union, St Petersburg, in 1996, applied to host the 2004 Summer Games, but the application did not make it to the short list considered by the International Olympic Committee (IOC). Notably, Putin had worked in St. Petersburg since 1991 and had held the position of Deputy Chairman of the City Government since 1994. However, Putin's biography when he worked in St Petersburg, from 1991 through 1996, is poorly documented and is considered among the "murkiest" periods of his life (Gessen, 2012). Any evidence of Putin's personal participation is extremely flimsy. Analyzing the failure of the project, for example, *New York Times* correspondent Steven Lee Myers, stated that Putin's boss, Anatoly Sobchak, was no longer the mayor when, in 1997, the IOC selected Athens as the host for the 2004 Summer Olympics, "having dropped St. Petersburg's bid hastily prepared with Putin's help" (Myers, 2015, p. 94).

PUTIN'S PERSONAL SPORT INTERESTS

Putin's connection to sports goes far beyond any of the previous leaders of Russia or the Soviet Union. For example, when applying for the 1980 Moscow Olympics, Soviet leader Leonid Brezhnev did not regard it as his personal project and even became alarmed about the expensive price tag, arguing for the cancellation of the Olympics at the last minute

(Tomilina, 2011). After the fall of the Soviet Union, Russian presidents began following the examples of their western counterparts by presenting themselves as athletic and skilled in sports. For example, President Yeltsin appeared in public playing tennis and popularized this sport in a country where there were few actual tennis courts.

Unlike Brezhnev, Putin tried to present the 2014 Sochi Olympics as his personal project reflecting his interest in sports, developing his image as a masculine and athletic leader (Sperling, 2014). Putin's official personal website describes his interests in several kinds of sport, but he is most closely associated with judo. "I was just a boy when I started judo. I became deeply interested in martial arts, their special philosophy, culture, relations with the opponent and the rules of combat," Putin stated on his personal website (Putin, n.d.). In 1976, Putin was Leningrad's judo champion. After graduating from Leningrad State University, Putin became a Master of Sports in judo. One Putin biographer even claimed that, until the fall of the Soviet Union, his judo club and the KGB were "the only important affiliation[s] that he had ever known" (Gessen, 2012).

After becoming president, Putin raised the prominence of judo in the same way that Yeltsin had backed tennis to promote his own image as a former judo star. The president's press secretary stressed that Putin personally supported the Russian National Judo Federation (Putin, 2012). The high level attention paid dividends after the Russian National Judo team appointed a new coach, Enzio Gamba, an Italian Olympic champion. After that, five out of six Russian competitors won medals during the 2012 London Summer Olympics. This achievement was all the more striking because Russia had never won in judo competitions before the 2012 London Olympics. Inspired by the achievements of the judo athletes, Putin visited one of the fights in London together with British Prime Minister David Cameron.

Putin considered the 2014 Olympics to be one of the country's top priorities after Russia won the bid to host the Winter Games in Sochi. He connected the Sochi Olympics directly with his name by personally attending the 2007 IOC meeting in Guatemala. After Putin addressed the IOC in English and French, the committee members voted to send the event to Russia.

INTERNATIONAL CHALLENGES FOR RUSSIA BEFORE THE OLYMPICS

The honor of hosting the Olympics is a challenge and opportunity for the host country, which must be ready for a number of unexpected, if inevitable, domestic and foreign challenges. Criticisms and controversy accompany the run-up to every Olympic contest. The 2012 London Olympics, for example, faced environmentalist challenges. China withstood intense pressure from international nongovernmental organizations before the start of the 2008 Beijing Olympics due to a number of human rights violations in the country. The 2004 Athens Olympics went through financial difficulties. In 2002, a member of the IOC suggested that the Winter Games be relocated from Salt Lake City, since the United States was a country at war with the Taliban in Afghanistan. Earlier, in 1980, U.S. President Jimmy

Carter asked the IOC to move the Olympic Games from Moscow after the Soviet invasion of Afghanistan.

As Russia sought to showcase its world-class athletes, culture, and economic development in Sochi, demonstrating its increasingly high international profile, it ran into trouble because the international spotlight exposed the authoritarian drift of its domestic policies and an array of unresolved issues. No doubt, some foreign countries and NGOs sought to capitalize on the globalized nature of the Olympic Games to urge the Kremlin to change the way that it dealt with troublesome topics, from the Russian occupation of Georgian territories to LGBT rights and the scandal surrounding asylum-seeker Edward Snowden. What patterns emerged in the Kremlin's responses to major issues and challenges? How did the Kremlin handle increasing domestic pressure and global scrutiny as the Games drew closer?

Kremlin Policies toward Post-Soviet Countries

Moscow has gained a reputation for pursuing an aggressive foreign policy in the post-Soviet space. There were many cases during the years following 1991 when Russia preyed on the weaknesses of its neighbors, using all kinds of instruments from trade sanctions to actual military invasion. But how did Moscow itself react to a neighbor's attempts at coercion? The case of the 2014 Olympics demonstrated that the Kremlin stood firm against such threats.

Russia faced many unresolved issues in the post-Soviet space, many of which could have escalated rapidly during the short timeframe leading up to the Olympics. Among the simmering conflicts were Russian diaspora problems in the Baltic states, political pressures in Moldova and breakaway Transnistria, Russian-Georgian relations in light of Russia's support for Abkhazian and South Ossetian separatists, relations with Armenia and Azerbaijan as they remained mired in a frozen conflict, the U.S. military transit center in Kyrgyzstan, tension in Russian-Ukrainian relations, and the new Eurasian Customs Union regulations. In fact, most post-Soviet states had some conflict with Russia and could use a boycott of the Games as a lever to pressure Moscow.

Yet, political tensions between Russia and its neighbors remained disconnected from the Olympic spirit. Perhaps one of the most eloquent examples of this was when Georgian President Mikheil Saakashvili was the first to congratulate Vladimir Putin when Russia won its Olympic bid in 2007. Tbilisi's initial enthusiasm did not soften Moscow's position over Russian-Georgian relations, however. In spite of the fact that Sochi was located close to the Georgian border, Russia did not hesitate to declare war against Georgia in August 2008. Then, rubbing salt into the wound after its victory in the five days of hostilities, the Kremlin recognized the independence of Abkhazia and South Ossetia, leading Tbilisi to use the Olympics as a platform to garner international attention in condemnation of Moscow's actions. With the support of some U.S. politicians, Georgia applied in vain to the IOC in September 2008 requesting that the Games not be held in Sochi. Then, Tbilisi declared it would not send Georgian athletes to participate. Proving its determination, Tbilisi also boycotted the Women's World Chess Championship in the Russian city of Nalchik in 2008 (despite projections that the Georgians were the favorites to win). In another move, in May

2011, Georgia recognized as genocide the 1864 Tsarist Russian mass murder of Circassians in Sochi, the last capital of independent Circassia.

During a September 2008 press conference, one month after the August war, Putin formulated the Kremlin's uncompromising policy toward the challenge of an Olympic boycott, saying, "If they do it once, it will destroy the entire structure of the Olympic movement.... However, on the other hand, if they want to take [the Sochi Games away], let them take on this burden" ("Putin: Khotiat utashchit' u nas Olimpiadu - pust' tashchat," 2008). Ultimately, the August 2008 war, the Russian occupation of Georgian territory next to Sochi, the multi-year UN resolutions against Russia, and the recognition of Sochi as a territory where genocide had been committed did not move the IOC to change its decision to hold the Olympics in Sochi. The committee's stubborn support for Russia was not surprising. In the past, the IOC had tolerated greater controversies: it did not move the 1980 Moscow Games in spite of the USSR's invasion of Afghanistan and the ensuing mass boycotts, nor did it shift the 1984 Los Angeles Games, which were boycotted by the USSR and its allies.

The firmness with which the Kremlin addressed the Georgian challenge prevented similar challenges from other post-Soviet states that might have been tempted to exert the same kind of pressure in their complicated relations with Russia. It became obvious that it would not affect the Olympics if, say, Kyiv, Chisinau, or Baku were to provoke the Russian military in Sevastopol, Transnistria, or Nagorno-Karabakh, or lead to any gains for Estonia if it joined Georgia in recognizing the Circassian genocide.

Ultimately, in 2013, Tbilisi changed its position and announced that Georgia would not boycott the 2014 Olympics. The shift in Tbilisi's policy followed the election of a new government. The Georgian case provides a remarkable example of how the same country tried to use the same political instrument three times, first supporting the Olympics in 2007, then deciding to boycott in 2008, and finally resolving to participate in 2013. Tbilisi's political flip-flops strikingly contrasted with Moscow's consistent line not to let its post-Soviet neighbors play the Olympic card.

Kremlin Policies with the West: Stopping Short of the Point of No Return

Russian policy toward Western states incorporated a much higher level of restraint and flexibility than Russia exhibited in its relations with the post-Soviet states. Russian-British relations before the Olympics were an example of this kind of discontinuous rapport. In 2006 there was high bilateral tension between Russia and the UK due to the assassination of former Russian spy Alexander Litvinenko, who had sought refuge in London. But in 2013, relations were stable even though the UK supported the Magnitsky list, an act of Congress that sought to punish Russians responsible for the prison death of a Russian lawyer who exposed hundreds of millions of dollars worth of corruption (Quinn & Aldrick, 2013). Generally, Moscow rarely applied to the West the same wide range of consistently harsh policies it used with the post-Soviet states, namely economic sanctions and military threats. When it came to threats from Western states, Moscow typically sought to challenge through "symmetric responses." In such a sensitive issue as a possible boycott of the 2014 Olympics, the Kremlin restrained itself from such policies, choosing not to cross certain "red lines" or "points of no return" in the escalation of crises.

Russia's policy towards the United States was less risk averse than its approach to Europe, with the Kremlin edging close to a point of no return. A series of confrontations brought the U.S. threat of Olympic boycott to the fore. The first U.S. boycott threat emerged in September 2008 as a reaction to the Russian-Georgian war, when U.S. Representatives Allyson Schwartz (D-PA) and Bill Shuster (R-PA), co-chairs of the House Georgia Caucus, introduced Congressional Resolution No. 412 ("No Russian Olympics in 2014") calling on the IOC to strip Russia of the 2014 Winter Olympics and to find a more suitable alternative location (Schwartz, 2008). At the time, however, the "reset" policy initiated by the Obama administration to improve ties with Russia made the idea of a boycott politically irrelevant.

Between 2008 and 2013, there were no discussions in the US of boycotting the Sochi Olympics. In 2013, however, the threat of a U.S. boycott again emerged during the scandal connected with Edward Snowden. On July 16, Sen. Lindsey Graham (R-SC) suggested that the United States should boycott the Olympics if Russia granted Snowden asylum, but Graham found little support among his colleagues in Washington or more broadly within the American public (Goyette, 2013). The senator's position did not alarm the Kremlin because even the more popular 2008 initiative in the U.S. Congress to boycott the Olympics had no consequences. Public opinion, however, shifted as the Snowden controversy dragged on and even more so as Russia's restrictive laws regarding sexual minorities attracted greater attention. The Kremlin miscalculated the White House's outlook when instead of relieving Russia-U.S. tensions from converging controversies, it escalated them by granting Snowden asylum. President Barack Obama responded by cancelling his planned meeting with Putin and, for the first time, referred to an Olympic boycott. The U.S. president went so far as to negatively describe Putin as behaving "like a bored kid" (Holland & Chadbourn, 2013). Even though Obama announced his personal position as against the boycott, the very fact that he referenced it demonstrated that the Kremlin had pushed him to the brink.

Feeling this, Moscow went silent and did not further escalate bilateral tensions. According to the Kremlin's "symmetric response" policy, one would expect Putin to do something in response to the cancellation of the summit and "cancel" something. At its red line, the Kremlin did not cancel the 2013 meeting between the U.S. Secretaries of State and Defense, John Kerry and Chuck Hagel, and the Russian Ministers of Foreign Affairs and Defense, Sergey Lavrov and Sergey Shoigu, which the U.S. Department of State then framed as generally productive (Shanker & Gordon, 2013).

On the social level, after the Russian parliament adopted laws banning "propaganda of nontraditional sexual relations" and blasphemy, the LGBT community and social activists in the United States, Europe, and elsewhere made anti-Olympic statements to which the Kremlin quickly responded with a statement assuring that there will be no persecution of LGBT athletes during the 2014 Olympics (President of Russia, 2013). European politicians also distanced themselves from any anti-Olympic activists. The Russian parliament that had been energetically adopting anti-gay laws abruptly became quiet. Though they did not

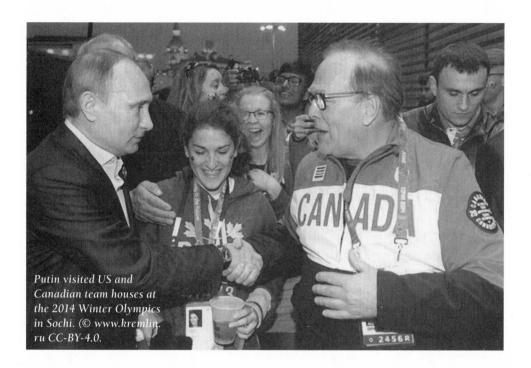

Putin visited US and Canadian team houses at the 2014 Winter Olympics in Sochi. (© www.kremlin. ru CC-BY-4.0.

go so far as to undo the laws, Russian officials explained that these laws were not against the LGBT community, but against encouraging so-called "untraditional sex" among minors, trying to show that there was some fine line that had not been crossed. In their statements and interviews, many Russian officials, including Putin, were quick to assure the international community that there would be no danger to gay athletes during the Games (Radia, 2014). In an interview with the Associated Press in September 2013, Putin, for the first time, expressed his readiness to meet with representatives of the LGBT community, which many experts interpreted as a result of pressure by LGBT athletes and the community in the West ("Putin Ready To Meet Gay Community Representatives," 2013).

Before the 2014 Sochi Olympics, the Games were treated as diplomatic capital. Such a tool was even used multiple times, as Georgia did when it announced in 2008 its intentions to boycott the Olympics and later in 2013 when it used the Games to restore relations with Russia. The Kremlin, for its part, became hostage to the Olympics, as it dealt with challenges of negative publicity and possible boycotts. With lasting tensions and new unexpected challenges, Russia several times came close to provoking different countries to boycott the Games. However, in the end, it navigated this uphill course with a firm hand toward neighbors like Georgia and more flexibility with the West. Ultimately, no country boycotted the Games. But, even if a boycott had taken place, it would not have been a fatal blow to the Kremlin, and the Games would have gone on.

MILITARY AND TERRORIST CHALLENGES FOR THE 2014 WINTER OLYMPICS

The preparations for the Olympics evolved through three distinct phases marked by different domestic and international security and diplomatic measures. At the beginning, the Kremlin assumed that Russia had achieved stability in the North Caucasus and implied that the Olympics would be open to everybody, including migrant workers who sought employment building Olympic facilities in the years before the opening ceremonies. Planners drew up the first security concept of the Games and construction plans in May 2007, a time when the Chechen insurgency seemed to have been defeated and its leaders were either dead or in hiding. The Kremlin elite considered the Chechen problem solved and did not anticipate other serious threats to stability in the region. They described the stabilization of Chechnya as a result of Putin's ability to take and centralize power, thus allowing Russia's return to the world stage (Wills & Moore, 2008). The organizers were sure that no serious domestic and international challenges faced Sochi. While applying for the right to hold the Olympics in 2007, the organizers specifically mentioned in the candidature file, "To date, there have been no recorded incidents of domestic or international terrorist acts in Sochi" (Sochi 2014, 2007, p. 29).

The emergence of the Caucasus Emirate, a terrorist organization operating in the North Caucasus region, forced changes in the Kremlin's domestic policy. To separate Sochi administratively from the restive North Caucasus region, the Kremlin carved a new North Caucasus federal district from the existing Southern federal district.

In October 2007, several months after Russia won the right to hold the Olympics, the leader of the Chechen insurgency, Doku Umarov, proclaimed his intention to establish an Islamic state, the Caucasus Emirate, which would include the entire Caucasus in addition to Chechnya (Moore, 2010; Moore & Tumelty, 2009). His grievances were rooted in domestic issues, and while foreign jihadists were able to participate in the fighting, their role was declining since its heyday between 1999 and 2002 (Moore & Tumelty, 2008). Russia's leaders did not try to address the root causes of the problem but sought to suppress the groups they dubbed "bandits" through a combination of repression and cooption (disbursing large sums of money). Hence terrorism in the area was "fueled and fostered by corruption that has acquired grotesque forms" (Baev, 2010). While regional leaders worried about the threats raised by these groups, the Kremlin did not employ special measures to secure the Olympic venues from 2007 through 2009, hoping that the combination of repression and cooption would be sufficient.

On the international stage, the unresolved territorial dispute between Georgia and the separatist regions of Abkhazia and South Ossetia, not far from Sochi, did not prevent Russia from winning the right to hold the Olympics in 2007. When Russia submitted its application to host the Olympics, the organizers did not specify that Russia might encounter any international threats. The application did not mention any particular military challenges except threats from domestic terrorist organizations. The 2008 Russian–Georgian war changed

Russia's international position, bringing it into open hostilities with a neighbor, and affected the preparations for the Games.

In the context of a complicated post-conflict relationship between the states, the Kremlin became worried about the Georgian threat to the security of the 2014 Sochi Olympics, reasoning that since Georgia had started a war during the 2008 Beijing Summer Olympics, it might do the same during the 2014 Sochi Winter Olympics. After the 2008 conflict, the Kremlin particularly feared NATO support for Georgia. In January 2012, Putin said that if NATO put a missile defense complex in Georgia, Russia would have no choice but to point its missiles "toward Georgian territory" ("Putin: Rossiia obespokoena vozmozhnostiu razmesheniia PRO SShA v Gruzii" ["Putin: Russia Is Concerned About the Possibility that the United States Will Place Missile Defense Systems in Georgia"], 2012). But the Kremlin regarded Georgia, with or without NATO support, as a threat. In February 2011, President Dmitry Medvedev stated that Russia has "certain problems with its neighbor Georgia" concerning the Sochi Olympics and ordered the security forces to prevent any pre-Olympic provocation ("Medvedev trebuet ne dopustit provokatsii pered olimpiadoi-2014" ["Medvedev Demands That There Be No Provocations Before the 2014 Olympiad"], 2011). On the other hand, Russia tried to work indirectly with NATO members, though such cooperation never went beyond a few meetings. In July 2011, a NATO-Russia meeting was held in Sochi, after which First Deputy Prime Minister Dmitry Kozak, who was overseeing Olympic preparations, said, "It seemed to me that the representatives of the NATO member countries were positively impressed" ["Kozak: Osnashenie rossiiskikh spetssluzb vpechatlilo NATO"], 2011). In October 2011, another forum in Sochi gathered the secret services of ten countries ("Spetssluzhby 10 stran obsudili bezopasnost OI-2014 v Sochi" ["The Special Services of Ten Countries Discussed the Security of the Olympic Games in Sochi"], 2011). In November 2011, Russia and Interpol reached an agreement that Interpol would provide security for the 2014 Olympics ("Spetssluzhby 10 stran obsudili bezopasnost OI-2014 v Sochi" ["The Special Services of Ten Countries Discussed the Security of the Olympic Games in Sochi"], 2011). At the same time, there were few signs of direct engagement by foreign security services in the preparations for the 2014 Olympics, and foreign secret services had no more access to the Games than foreign journalists—that is, limited and under the strict control of the Russian secret services.

Faced with increasing international and domestic challenges, toward the end of 2009, the Kremlin understood that it could not secure the entire region. The Kremlin therefore imposed territorial-administrative changes in the North Caucasus and separated the greater Sochi area from the center of destabilization in the North Caucasus republics by dividing the Southern federal district, which until then had included both Sochi and the restive North Caucasus region. In May 2010, Russian President Dmitry Medvedev issued a decree: "On Providing Security During the Twenty-Second Winter Olympic Games and Eleventh Paralympic Games of 2014 in Sochi" ("Ukaz Prezidenta RF ot 14.05.2010 No. 594 'Ob obespechenii bezopasnosti pri provedenii XXII Olimpiiskikh zimnikh igr i XI Paralimpiiskikh zimnikh igr 2014 goda v Sochi'" [Decree of the RF President of May 14, 2010, no. 594, "On

Supplying Security During the Conduct of the Twenty-Second Olympic Winter Games and the Eleventh Paralympic Winter Games in 2014 in Sochi"], 2010). The practical impact of Medvedev's decree was that Russia launched military and antiterror preparations for the Olympics, including military drills on the Black Sea, along Russia's borders, and in the Caucasus Mountains. The Kremlin prioritized counterintelligence security over antiterrorism security, behaving as if it was more afraid of a foreign threat than any violence from inside the country (Soldatov, Borogan, & Walker, 2013).

HUMAN RIGHT VIOLATIONS AND THE 2014 OLYMPICS

Putin personally supervised the Olympic preparations during their last year. In February 2013, he announced that he was dealing with Olympic issues on a daily basis, an unprecedented level of engagement in the Olympic process for a national leader ("'Vykhodnykh ne byvaet': Putin prinyal v Sochi vpechatlennogo stroitel'stvom Yanukovicha," 2013 [Working without weekends: Putin met, in Sochi, with Yanukivich who was impressed by the building progress]). In May 2013, Putin confirmed again that he was working on the Olympics every day (ibid). The president's personal involvement in the megaproject showed not only his interest in sports, but also the Kremlin's lack of capability to create an effective mechanism to prepare the Olympics without the president's constant oversight and intervention.

Putin's personal involvement during the last year of preparations for the Olympics might have hardened the organizers' policies toward the migrant workers who were helping to construct the facilities Sochi required. Though Putin never mentioned his participation in planning sports events during his work as Deputy Chairman of the St Petersburg City Government, he might have used some of the methods of that time during the 2014 Olympics. In July, 1994, St. Petersburg hosted the Goodwill Games and the city government drove "unwanted migrant workers out of the city before the games opened" (Myers, 2015, p. 93).

In 2007, however, the Olympic organizers stated in their application that Sochi itself was a safe and secure environment: "Sochi is a diverse, multicultural city with more than four hundred thousand inhabitants representing more than a hundred nationalities who welcome almost four million tourists each year" (Sochi 2014, 2007, p. 25). The organizers initially announced their intention to attract many foreign workers and Russian citizens from other regions to help prepare for the Olympics. Initial estimates suggested that about two hundred thousand migrant workers would take part (Naumov, 2009). In practice, however, the organizers isolated Sochi from foreigner and nonethnic Russians to the point where, officially, only 12,959 workers from other Russian regions and 7,339 foreigners worked on the Olympic facilities in 2011 (Chelokian, 2011; Naumov, 2008). Most of the migrant workers arrived from former Soviet republics, including Uzbekistan, Ukraine, Belarus, Moldova, Tajikistan, and Kyrgyzstan. It was easier for citizens of the former Soviet republics to find work in Sochi because they did not need visas and could stay in Russia for ninety days, sufficient time to obtain a work permit. Workers from other countries, like Turkey and Serbia, mostly came by special invitation from the Olympic organizers. Although Putin met with

Turkish Prime Minister Recep Tayyip Erdogan in May 2009 and agreed to welcome Turkish workers to the facilities, heightened security precautions made their arrival difficult and only 546 Turks worked at the Olympic facilities in 2011 (Naumov, 2009).

Whereas, during 2007–2010, Russia advertised liberal and easy conditions to register and work on Olympic facilities in Sochi, the deportation of foreign workers became popular after 2010. In 2011, 154 foreign workers were deported. Many workers also faced fines. In 2011, the courts ordered foreign workers in Sochi to pay 31,727,250 rubles (more than $1 million); informally, they may have paid much more due to the extensive corruption in Russian society (Chelokian, 2011). In 2013, the authorities registered 24,000 violations of migration law, including 4,000 violations by law enforcement agencies, and deported 3,000 foreign workers from the Krasnodar region, with half coming from Sochi ("Aleksandr Tkachev potreboval ubrat' iz Sochi vsekh nelegalov cherez dva mesiatsa," 2013 [Alexandr Tkachev demanded to remove all illegal immigrants from Sochi within two months]).

In 2013, *Human Rights Watch* reported many violations of the rights of migrant workers in Sochi (Human Rights Watch, 2013). Among the most prominent were employment without a contract, failure to provide sufficient accommodation for employees, and failure to pay full salaries on time. Workers who complained about these abuses were often deported from Russia.

In the run-up to the Olympics, the level of xenophobia increased in Russian society. In 2009, about 52% of Russians expressed negative attitudes against foreign workers migrating to Russia, but by 2013, the figure increased to 78% ("Levada-tsentr: Pochti 80% rossiian - protiv pritoka migrantov," 2013 [Almost 80% of Russians are against the increase of immigrants]). Given those numbers, the Putin government probably had strong popular support for its eviction of the foreign workers. However, the shabby treatment of the workers hurt Russia's image in the Caucasus and Central Asia countries that had sent the workers to Russia in order to make a living.

THE SOCHI OLYMPICS AND RUSSIAN ANNEXATION OF CRIMEA

In the Western media and policy-making community, the 2014 Russian invasion of Ukraine and annexation of Crimea, which took place immediately after the closing ceremonies, overshadowed the Sochi Olympics and prevented a proper analysis of the Olympic role in Russian domestic and international policy. The Kremlin's decision to invade a neighboring country seemed to contradict the Kremlin's decade-long, $50 billion effort to promote Russia's positive image on the international stage.

While the annexation of Crimea overshadowed the results of the Sochi Olympics for the West and caused Russia's international isolation, the Russian population viewed both events in terms of continuity rather than disjunction. The population saw them as part of the Kremlin's strategy of raising Russia "from its knees." According to that image, the new Russia rose from one knee by hosting the 2014 Sochi Olympics, the same way as the USSR hosted the 1980 Moscow Olympics, and instantly after that Russia also rose from its second knee by annexing Crimea, or according to the Kremlin's rhetoric, taking back territory that Russia unjustly lost after the fall of the USSR. Indeed, pairing the peaceful and aggressive events is highly profitable for the current regime in Russia.

The 2014 Sochi Olympics coincided with the anti-regime unrest in Ukraine and the flight of President Viktor Yanukovych to Russia. Because of Putin's prominent role in organizing the Olympics and annexation of Crimea, many experts questioned if there was a connection between these two events. While nobody doubted the Kremlin's involvement in both events, since Putin himself stressed his personal role in them, expert opinion varies widely on the question of whether the Kremlin used the Sochi Olympics as a tool for the annexation of Crimea.

Conspiratorially minded analysts claim that all the aforementioned events were part of a preplanned Kremlin plot. Though, before the Sochi Olympics, there were no accounts that the Kremlin had a plan to annex Crimea, some analysts have found signs that such plans existed. *Financial Times* Moscow correspondent Kathrin Hille reported retrospectively that "on the eve of the Winter Olympics, many Moscow intellectuals were struggling to get into a festive mood. Vague rumors were swirling in Russia's capital that President Vladimir Putin was planning some aggressive move and that after the games, "something terrible will happen" (Hille, 2014). She quotes Johan Lybeck, a former Swedish military intelligence officer specializing in Russia during the Cold War, who after the annexation of Crimea, developed a theory that the Kremlin planned before the Olympics to remove the Ukrainian president from power. With that task in mind, the Russian FSB infiltrated the Ukrainian Berkut riot police, and after Ukraine's new government disbanded the riot police, Berkut officers went to Crimea, seized the region's two airports and helped Russian paratroopers invade the peninsula. Another opinion is that the opportunity to annex Crimea appeared during the Games and the Kremlin used the resources gathered for the Olympics—concentrated security forces, popular patriotic sentiments, and infrastructure—to invade Crimea.

A careful analysis of the timeline of events suggests that the decision to invade Ukraine indeed was made during the Olympics. Before the launch of the opening ceremonies, the Kremlin announced that "Vladimir Putin will go to Sochi on February 4, in the run-up to the opening of the XXII Winter Olympic Games,"—that is, several days before the opening of the games that took place on February 7 ("Vladimir Putin will go to Sochi on February 4, in the run-up to the opening of the XXII Winter Olympic Games," 2014). Putin spent a week in Sochi, attending all kinds of PR activities. Once the actual Games began, Putin actually spent little time at the competition. After February 9th, Putin left Sochi and spent most of his time in Moscow, only briefly coming back to witness the sporting events.

Putin recalled in *Crimea. The Way Home* (2015), a documentary broadcast on Russian state-controlled television, that the decision to annex Crimea was made in the Kremlin on February 23, in the morning of the closing ceremony for the Winter Olympics, after the operation to save Ukrainian President Yanukovych from being captured by Ukrainian revolutionaries began. Putin stated in his interview for the film,

The operation [to save Yanukovych] began late on February 22 and ended around 7:00 am the next day. And I will not deny that as we were leaving, I told the four colleagues who were with me, "The latest developments in Ukraine force us to begin working on returning Crimea to Russia.". . . I gave them some instructions about what needed to be done. (Kondrashov, 2015).

Thus, before the 2014 Olympics were over, Russia's leader had made the decision to invade Crimea. The connection between these two events, however, remains unexplained. On one hand, the Kremlin spent more than $50 billion on the Olympics, aiming to improve Russia's international profile; on the other hand, Russia's reputation was dramatically damaged by the invasion in Crimea.

Though contradictory from an outsider's perspective, the Sochi Olympics and annexation of Crimea were logically connected from the Russian point of view. Both events were part of the Kremlin's narrative of restoring Russian greatness after the fall of the USSR; the 2014 Sochi Games matched the 1980 Moscow Games, and the annexation of Crimea brought back the "glory" of Stalin's annexations of new territories to the USSR before WWII. The opening ceremony provided additional context connecting Sochi and Crimea. The Kremlin shaped the Sochi Olympics and the invasion of Crimea in the same imperial cultural narrative. The opening ceremony portrayed Russia as an empire, emphasizing the glories of Russia's imperial history. Indeed, the opening ceremony portrayed Putin's Russia as equal to the Soviet Union at its height. Culturally, the imperial narrative of the opening ceremony of the Sochi Olympics matched the Kremlin's propaganda narrative of annexing Crimea as a step toward restoring the Russian Empire/USSR.

In practical terms, the Kremlin regarded annexation of Crimea as another megaproject, just like the Olympics had been. From a military perspective, the Kremlin's use of the unprecedented security forces accumulated during the Sochi Olympics partly explains why the Russian invasion into the nearby Crimean Peninsula was so effective. From an economic perspective, the organizers of the Sochi Olympics transferred their resources to Crimea. The Olympstroy state company, established by Putin to organize and execute the Olympic preparation, easily became Krymstroy, a new entity designed to oversee the Russian occupation of Crimea. From an administrative perspective, the Kremlin's curator of the Olympics, Dmitry Kozak, became the overseer of the new Crimean Republic and Sebastopol, its capital city. In terms of the media, after mobilizing all of its propaganda efforts around the Sochi Olympics, the Kremlin could easily deploy them in what it called an "information war" after the Crimean invasion.

The Olympics served and strengthened Putin's personal regime, with his popularity rising from 65%–69% during January–February, 2014, as the games unfolded. The even more dramatic rise of Putin's popularity among Russians after the annexation of Crimea showed that, in the opinion of Russian citizens, the military action did not contradict the narrative of the Olympics, which is devoted to peaceful competition. The Crimean invasion and annexation boosted Putin's support level to 80% in March and 84% in June 2014.

Later, the invasion of Ukraine lifted Putin's popularity in Russia even further, up to 87%, a rating similar to levels previously achieved after Russia's war in Georgia in 2005 (88%) and in Chechnya in 1999 (84%; Levada Analytical Center, 2014). The vast majority of Russians approved of both events as ways to improve the status of their country and strengthen the position of its unchallenged leader.

CONCLUSION

Putin saw the 2014 Sochi Olympics and other sport mega-events as useful in promoting his diplomatic efforts to demonstrate Russia's greatness on the world stage. Sporting mega-events attract a large international television audience and their production requires world-class infrastructure and sophisticated management skills. Any errors or oversights can result in embarrassing glitches seen by the entire world. China effectively used the 2008 Olympics to announce its arrival as a great power on the world stage and Putin saw Russia as achieving similar purposes with the 2014 Games.

However, Putin's use of such events has not been effective in winning Russia greater respect. Today, Russia's standing in global popular opinion is lower than it has ever been. Putin's poor handling of human rights turned the Sochi Olympics into a referendum on his values, and many world leaders boycotted the games even though athletes from their countries competed. In response to Putin's legislation against "gay propaganda," President Barak Obama, Germany's Angela Merkel, and numerous other Western leaders refused to attend the Olympics in Russia. The US instead sent a relatively low-level delegation that prominently featured members of the LGBT community, intending to deliver a sharp rebuke to Putin.

The ongoing fighting in Ukraine, prompting Western sanctions, not only undercut the dividends Russia hoped to receive from the Olympics, but it is threatening to undermine any diplomatic value that Russia hopes to generate from the next sport mega-event it will host—the 2018 World Cup. The U.S. decision to arrest key members of the FIFA leadership, and successfully pressure President Sepp Blatter to resign, similarly triggered fears among Russia's leadership that Western law enforcement agencies would try to expose Russian corruption in winning the right to host the 2018 soccer championship.

In the face of these diplomatic debacles, Putin's main audience for his mega-events is ultimately Russia's citizens, whom he is seeking to impress in order to maintain his grip on power. He was willing to spend $50 billion on the Sochi Games and many more billions on the World Cup in order to demonstrate to his constituents that he is capable of leading Russia at the forefront of the world's most important countries. Achieving such status gives Russians a source of pride and a feeling that Russia has achieved its rightful place regardless of what populations in the West actually think. Even though Russia is an authoritarian country, Putin needs to maintain popular support to be able to fend off potential challengers.

In fact, Russia's preparations for the sporting mega-events it hosts are part of the problem for its diplomacy. Russia is ranked as one of the most corrupt countries in the world.

The lavish sums it spent on the Olympics and World Cup, at a time when it is cutting back on pensions and other social support expenditures, call into question the real impact of Putin's leadership on his own country. While sports festivals are meant to bring the world's countries together for peaceful competition, in the case of Russia, they often further exacerbate existing tensions between Western democracies and their increasingly hostile neighbor.

DISCUSSION QUESTIONS

1. How can authoritarian leaders use the Olympic Games to boost their own power?

2. Why did the Soviet Union and then Russia attach so much importance to hosting the Olympic Games?

3. What was the role of Putin's personality and love of sport in Russia's decision to host the games?

4. Did hosting the Olympics improve Russia's international image?

5. Were the security preparations for the Sochi Olympics successful? Will their legacy have lasting consequences for Russia's political and economic system?

6. Did hosting the Olympics help Russia improve its human rights and environment situation?

7. What, if any, is the connection between the Olympics and Russia's decision to invade Ukraine and annex Crimea?

8. Were the Olympics a success from the point of view of Russia?

9. How will historians eventually view the 2014 Sochi Olympics in the context of games held in other countries?

10. What are the similarities and differences between the 2014 Sochi Olympics in Russia and 1980 Moscow Olympics in Soviet Union?

REFERENCES

Aleksandr Tkachev potreboval ubrat' iz Sochi vsekh nelegalov cherez dva mesiatsa [Aleksandr Tkachev demanded to remove all illegal immigrants from Sochi within two months]. (2013, November 9). Blogsochi. [Weblog]. Retrieved from http://blogsochi.ru/content/aleksandr-tkachev-potreboval-ubrat-iz-sochi-vsekh-nelegalov-cherez-dva-mesyatsa

Alt, H., & Alt, E. (1964). *The new Soviet man, his upbringing and character development.* New York, NY: Bookman Associates.

Baev, P. K. (2010, October). The terrorism–corruption nexus in the North Caucasus. *PONARS Eurasia Policy Memo, 114.* Retrieved from http://www.ponarseurasia.org/node/5215

Chelokian, A. (2011, December 5). Migratsionnyi bum po-Sochinski [Migration boom Sochi style]. *Infotsentr 2014.* Retrieved from http://infocenter2014.ru/events/publications/publications_3712.html

Constitutional Federal Law of 25 December 2000. On the State Anthem of the Russian Federation. Website of the Constitution of the Russian Federation, http://constitution.garant.ru/act/base/182785/

Edelman, R. (1993). *Serious fun: A history of spectator sports in the USSR.* New York, NY: Oxford University Press.

Gessen, M. (2012). *The man without a face: The unlikely rise of Vladimir Putin.* New York, NY: Riverhead Books.

Goyette, B. (2013, July 16). Lindsey Graham: Boycott 2014 Olympics if Russia gives Snowden asylum. *The Huffington Post*. Retrieved from http://www.huffingtonpost.com/2013/07/16/lindsey-graham-boycott-olympics-snowden_n_3607528.html

Hille, K. (2014, March 2). Russia watchers say military manoeuvre was long in the making. *Financial Times*. Retrieved from http://www.ft.com/intl/cms/s/0/3a8833b6-a230-11e3-87f6-00144feab7de.html#axzz3jHa07ybK

Hobsbawm, E. (1990). *Nations and nationalisms since 1780: Programme, myth, reality*. Cambridge, UK: Cambridge University Press.

Holland, S., & Chadbourn, M. (2013, August 9). Obama describes Putin as 'like a bored kid'. Reuters. Retrieved from http://www.reuters.com/article/2013/08/09us-usa-russia-obama-idUSBRE9780XS20130809

Human Rights Watch. (2013). *Russia: Migrant Olympic workers cheated, exploited*. New York, NY: Human Rights Watch.

Kavokin, A., & Evstifeev, O. (2015, April 15). Zharkie. Letnie. Nepiterskie: Plyusy i Minusy Provedeniia Olimpiiskikh Igr v Peterburge [Hot. Cool. Non-Petersburgish: Advantages and disadvantages for holding Olympic games at St. Petersburg]. *Sport den' za dnem*. Retrieved from http://www.sportsdaily.ru/articles/zharkie-letnie-nepiterskie

Kondrashov, A. (2015, March 15). Krym. Put' na Rodinu [Crimea. The way home]. *Rossiia 24*. Retrieved from https://www.youtube.com/watch?v=t42-71RpRgI

Kozak: Osnashenie rossiiskikh spetssluzb vpechatlilo NATO [Kozak: The Russian special service's equipment impressed NATO]. (2011, July 4). *Vzgliad*. Retrieved from http://www.vz.ru/news/2011/7/4/504710.html

Lamtsov, M. A. (1989, September 23). Nashe Interview. Budet Li Sochi Stolitsei Olimpiady? [Our interview: Will Sochi become an Olympic Capital?] *Argumenty i Fakty*. Retrieved from http://www.aif.ru/archive/1650835

Levada-tsentr: Pochti 80% rossiian - protiv pritoka migrantov [Almost 80% of Russians are against the increase of immigrants]. (2013, November 5). *Fontanka*. Retrieved from http://www.fontanka.ru/2013/11/05/047/

Levada Analytical Center. (2014). Approval of Putin. Retrieved from http://www.levada.ru/eng/indexes-0

Makarychev, A. (2013). Rossiiskie olimpiiskie diskursy: Effekty unifikatsii i mnogoobrazia [Russian Olympic discourses: Effects of unification and diversity]. *Neprikosnovennyi Zapas*, 2(88), 86-100.

Medvedev trebuet ne dopustit' provokatsii pered olimpiadoi-2014. [Medvedev demands that there be no provocations before the 2014 Olympiad]. (2011, February 18). *RIA Novosti*. Retrieved from http://ria.ru/society/20110218/335730959.html

Moore, C. (2010). *Contemporary violence: Postmodern war in Kosovo and Chechnya*. Manchester, UK: Manchester University Press.

Moore, C., & Tumelty, P. (2008). Foreign fighters and the case of Chechnya: A critical assessment. *Studies in Conflict and Terrorism, 31*, 412–433.

Moore, C., & Tumelty, P. (2009). Assessing unholy alliances in Chechnya: From communism and nationalism to Islamism and Salafism. *Journal of Communist Studies and Transition Politics, 25*, 73-94.

Myers, S. L. (2015). *The new tsar: The rise and reign of Vladimir Putin*. New York, NY: Alfred A. Knopf.

Naumov, I. (2008, July 4). Ekologi oderzhali pervuyu pobedu na sochinskoi Olimpiade. *Nezavisimaya gazeta*. Retrieved from http://www.ng.ru/economics/2008-07-04/4_ecology.html

Naumov, I. (2009, June 18). Sochi zastroiat inostrantsy [Foreigners are building Sochi]. *Nezavisimaia gazeta*. Retrieved from www.ng.ru/economics/2009-06-18/4_Sochi.html

Nemtsov, B., & Martynyuk, L. (2013, December 6). Winter Olympics in the sub-tropics: Corruption and abuse in Sochi. *The Interpreter.* Retrieved from http://www.interpretermag.com/winter-olympics-in-the-sub-tropics-corruption-and-abuse-in-sochi/

Persson, E., & Petersson, B. (2013). "Political mythmaking and the 2014 Winter Olympics in Sochi: Olympism and the Russian great power myth." *East European Politics 30,* 192-209.

President of Russia. (2013, 30 June). Vneseny izmeneniia v zakon o zashchite detei ot informatsii, prichiniaiushchei vred ikh zdorov'iu i razvitiu [Amendments have been made to the Law on the protection of children from information harmful to their health and development]. Retrieved from http://kremlin.ru/acts/18423

Putin Ready To Meet Gay Community Representatives. (2013, September 4). *RFE/RL.* Retrieved from http://www.rferl.org/content/russia-putin-ready-to-meet-gay-representatives/25095927.html

Putin, V. (no date). Personal Website. Interests. http://en.putin.kremlin.ru/interests

Putin, V. (2005). Annual Address to the Federal Assembly of the Russian Federation on August, 25, 2005. *Official website of the President of Russia.* Retrieved from http://en.kremlin.ru/events/president/transcripts/22931

Putin, V. (2012, August 3). Putin smotrit sorevnovaniya i sam zanimetsya bor'boi [Putin watches the sport competition and wrestles himself]. *RIA-Novosti.* Retrieved from http://ria.ru/sport/20120803/715525262.html

Putin: Khotiat utashchit' u nas Olimpiadu - pust' tashchat. (2008, February 9) [Putin: If they want to take away from us the Olympics – let them take it away]. Rosbalt. Retrieved from http://www.rosbalt.ru/main/2008/09/02/519818.html

Putin: Rossiia obespokoena vozmozhnostiu razmeshcheniia PRO SShA v Gruzii [Putin: Russia is concerned about the possibility that the United States will place missile defense systems in Georgia]. (2012, January 18). *RIA Novosti.* Retrieved from http://ria.ru/defense_safety/20120118/542707064.html

Quinn, J., & Aldrick, P. (2013, July 8). Russians linked to Sergei Magnitsky case banned from entering UK. *The Telegraph.* Retrieved from http://www.telegraph.co.uk/finance/financial-crime/10167401/Russians-linked-to-Sergei-Magnitsky-case-banned-from-entering-UK.html

Radia, K. (2014, January 19). Vladimir Putin defends anti-gay law, but vows no Problems' for Olympic visitors. *ABC News.* Retrieved from http://abcnews.go.com/International/vladimir-putin-defends-anti-gay-law-vows-problems/story?id=21588617

Schwartz, R. A. (2008, September 19). Members of Congress announce "No Russian Olympics in 2014". *Legistorm.* Retrieved from http://www.legistorm.com/stormfeed/view_rss/273815/member/465.html

Shanker, T., & Gordon, M. R. (2013, August 9). Kerry and Hagel meet with their Russian counterparts. *New York Times.* Retrieved from http://www.nytimes.com/2013/08/10/world/europe/kerry-and-hagel-meet-with-their-russian-counterparts.html

Sochi 2014. (2007). Sochi Candidature File. Retrieved from http://web.archive.org/web/20100103043040/http://sochi2014.com/sch_questionnaire

Soldatov, A., Borogan, I., & Walker, S. (2013, October 6). As Sochi Olympic venues are built, so are Kremlin's surveillance networks. *The Guardian.* Retrieved from www.theguardian.com/world/2013/oct/06/sochi-olympicvenues-kremlin-surveillance

Sperling, V. (2014). *Sex, politics, and Putin: Political legitimacy in Russia.* Oxford, UK: Oxford University Press.

Spetssluzhby 10 stran obsudili bezopasnost' OI-2014 v Sochi [The Special Services of Ten Countries Discussed the Security of the Olympic Games in Sochi]. (2011, October 28). RIA Novosti. Retrieved from http://sport.ria.ru/olympic_games/20111028/473548744.html

Tomilina, N. G. (2011). *Piat' kolets pod kremlevskimi zvezdami: Dokumental'naia khronika olimpi-ady-80 v Moskve* [Five rings under the Kremlin stars: Documented chronicles of 1980 Olympics in Moscow]. Moscow, Russia: Mezhdunarodnyi fond "Demokratiia."

Ukaz Prezidenta RF ot 14.05. (2010). No. 594 Ob obespechenii bezopasnosti pri provedenii XXII Olimpiiskikh zimnikh igr i XI Paralimpiiskikh zimnikh igr 2014 goda v Sochi [Decree of the RF president of May 14, 2010, no. 594, "On supplying security during the conduct of the twenty-second Olympic Winter Games and the Eleventh Paralympic Winter Games in 2014 in Sochi]. (2010, May 15). Russian president's Website. Retrieved from http://graph.document.kremlin.ru/page.aspx?1;1263337

Vladimir Putin will go to Sochi on February 4, in the run-up to the opening of the XXII Winter Olympic Games. (2014, February 4). *Kremlin.ru*. Retrieved from http://en.kremlin.ru/events/president/news/20137

Vykhodnykh ne byvaet: Putin prinyal v Sochi vpechatlennogo stroitel'stvom Yanukovicha [Working without weekends: Putin met, in Sochi, with Yanukivich who was impressed by the building progress]. (2013, 26 May). *Newsru.com*. Retrieved from http://www.newsru.com/russia/26may2013/sochi.html

Wills, D., & Moore, C. (2008). Securitising the Caucasus: From political violence to place branding in Chechnya. *Place Branding and Public Diplomacy, 4*, 252–262.

Yeltsin, B. (1991, July 11). Presidential Inauguration speech on July 10, 1991. *Rossiiskaia gazeta*.

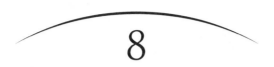

8

BUILDING STADIUMS, BUILDING BRIDGES: GEOPOLITICAL STRATEGY IN CHINA

TIMOTHY KELLISON · ALICIA CINTRON

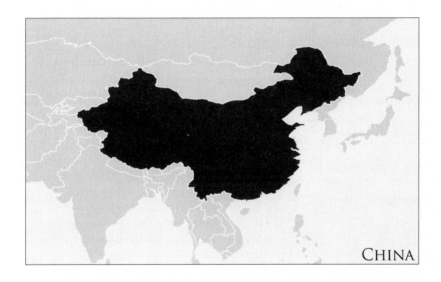

For 60 years, the People's Republic of China has championed the practice of so-called *stadium diplomacy*, in which the cost to construct or renovate a sports stadium in an emerging nation–state is subsidized wholly or in large part by a sponsoring state (Will, 2011, 2012). To date, China has provided support for more than 85 indoor and outdoor stadiums across Africa, Asia, Latin America and the Caribbean, and the South Pacific (Information Office of the State Council, 2011). These facilities range in size (from a 1,000-seat recreational complex in the Cook Islands to 60,000-seat stadia in Kenya and Senegal) and scope (from serving citizens and holding local matches to hosting major international events such as the Cricket World Cup and Africa Cup of Nations). Despite variations in function, each stadium is meant to symbolize unity between its state and China. For example, separate venues in Gabon and Benin are each named Stade de l'Amitié (Friendship Stadium; Ross, 2014). Additionally, at Mozambique's Estádio Nacional do Zimpeto, a plaque declares, "The friendship between China and Mozambique will last forever like the heavens and the earth" (Ross, 2014, para. 10).

China's stadium diplomacy represents a small part—less than 5% of all projects—of a comprehensive foreign aid program that includes agriculture, public facilities, infrastructure, and industry (Information Office of the State Council, 2011). Still, given the visibility of and meaningfulness attached to sports facilities (Kellison & Mondello, 2012). China has been able to leverage its support of stadium construction abroad for a number of benefits. While at least part of China's international stadium policy aims to grow its national economy (e.g., through revenues generated by loan and interest repayment), it has also facilitated the formation of diplomatic ties with strategic allies. For example, stadium partnerships with states rich in natural resources, such as Ecuador and Angola, have improved China's access to oil (Guest, 2009). Chinese stadium diplomacy has also been used to raise the state's profile against its competitors. At a time when the United States has cut its foreign aid program significantly, China has increased spending in Latin America and the Caribbean (Will, 2012). Stadium diplomacy has also been used as leverage in China–Taiwan relations. For instance, after cutting diplomatic ties with Taiwan, Costa Rica received over US$800 million in bonds and loans from China (Wilson, 2014).

In this chapter, we chronicle China's use of sport as a tool of geopolitical strategy. First, we provide background on China's general foreign aid policies, including its origins and forms. Next, we explore several examples of China's outward stadium investments, including developments in Africa, the Caribbean, Central America, and the South Pacific. We conclude the chapter by considering the possible reasons that underlie China's financial and economic support of stadium development overseas. As introduced in the section below, these motives may be at odds with China's official no-strings-attached policy.

CHINA'S FOREIGN AID AT LARGE

As one of the fastest growing economies worldwide, China has grown its international presence significantly over the past two decades, due in part to the government's relaxed oversight of outward direct investment (Wang, Mao, & Gou, 2014). While its foreign aid program has been criticized for a lack of transparency, China's central information office has outlined several forms of foreign assistance, including complete projects focusing on infrastructure and agriculture (the category likely representing sports stadiums), goods and materials, technical expertise, human resources development, medical assistance, volunteers and volunteer programs, humanitarian aid, and debt relief (Bräutigam, 2011; Grimm, 2011; Information Office of the State Council, 2014).

More broadly, China's foreign aid program aims to "improve people's livelihood" (i.e., by promoting agricultural development, improving education, enhancing medical and health services, building public welfare facilities, and providing humanitarian aid) and "promote economic and social development" (i.e., by improving infrastructure, strengthening capacity building, promoting trade partnerships, and bolstering environmental protection; Information Office of the State Council, 2014, p. 1). The aid packages themselves may include grants, loans (ranging from interest-free to those of low- or high-interest), lines of credit, and in-kind gifts or services (Bernal, 2015). Based on reports provided by the Chinese government, the majority of its foreign assistance (about 56%) is in the form of concessional loans, which are typically marked by below-market interest rates and/or extended grace periods (Information Office of the State Council, 2014; International Monetary Fund, 2014). Grants (36%) and interest-free loans (8%) represent the remaining pieces of China's foreign aid allocations.

Beijing's official position on its foreign aid program depicts a policy that supports collaborative partnership rather than quid pro quo trade:

> When providing foreign assistance, China adheres to the principles of not imposing any political conditions, not interfering in the internal affairs of the recipient countries, and fully respecting their right to independently choosing their own paths and models of development. The basic principles China upholds in providing foreign assistance are mutual respect, equality, keeping promises, mutual benefits, and win-win agreements. (Information Office of the State Council, 2014, p. 1)

On the other hand, critical analyses of China's foreign aid policies have—like critiques of other state's outward aid—speculated about its underlying intent, especially in cases of extremely generous economic gifting to developing states and emerging economies in Africa, South America, and the Caribbean. As noted by Bräutigam (2011), "critics generally believe that China's aid program is enormous and focused primarily on propping up pariah regimes or smoothing the way to Chinese companies to gain access to resources" (p. 753). As noted in Bernal's (2015) assessment of China–Caribbean partnerships, these foreign aid programs are likely a messy combination of several strategies: "The economic interaction... cannot be explained entirely by economic factors, but is best understood as an economic relationship embedded within a political and diplomatic relationship" (p. 1411). These myriad factors will be discussed further in a later section of this chapter.

A foundational aspect of China's international diplomacy centers on its longstanding conflict with Taiwan (i.e., cross-Strait relations). For example, throughout the process of allying with Caribbean nation–states, "China has been cognizant of its diplomatic rivalry with Taiwan" (Bernal, 2015, p. 1412). A suspected reason for China's historic interest in the Caribbean basin is the fact that a large number of states in this region share diplomatic relations with Taiwan, a direct violation of Beijing's "One China policy" (Alexander, 2011). Under this policy, China and Taiwan cannot be recognized as two separate states, leaving governments to choose between the People's Republic of China (China) and the Republic of China (Taiwan). The tension in cross-Strait relations dates back to the Chinese Revolution of 1949, when mainland China was claimed by the Communist China Party, leaving Kuomintang (Nationalist Party) to retreat to Taiwan (Office of the Historian, 2015). The importing of Chinese goods has grown worldwide, even in states that have not adopted a One China policy. Still, those states that have allied with China (either always or by breaking ties with Taiwan) have enjoyed greater economic cooperation and aid from Beijing, as illustrated in the next section.

STADIUM DIPLOMACY IN PRACTICE

A number of examples illustrate China's efforts to foster diplomatic and strategic alliances with other nation–states, including Tanzania (Amaan Stadium), Angola (Estádio 11 de Novembro, Estádio Nacional do Chiazi, Ombaka National Stadium, and Tundavala National Stadium), Jamaica (Sligoville Stadium), Antigua and Barbuda (Sir Vivian Richards Stadium), Costa Rica (National Stadium), Kiribati (Betia Sports Complex), and Laos (Lao National Stadium). These prominent Chinese-sponsored sports facilities are highlighted in turn below.

TANZANIA

The first foreign stadium construction project completed by the Chinese government was Amaan Stadium, a 15,000-seat venue constructed in 1970 in Zanzibar (Ross, 2014). Amaan Stadium has primarily been used to host football matches. Major renovations in 2010 allowed the stadium to host these matches during the day as well as under floodlights (Juma, 2013). The Chinese government provided ¥ 48 million (about US $7.5 million) for the renovations, which represented the stadium's first major overhaul since its opening ("Kudos to Karume," 2010; "SMZ to Protect Amaan Stadium," 2010). According to an editorial published in Tanzania's *Guardian,* these renovations were meant to reflect the continuing friendship between the two states ("Kudos to Karume," 2010). As further gestures of amity, the Chinese government donated a primary school to Zanzibar and provided anti-malaria drugs (Embassy of the People's Republican of China in the United Republic of Tanzania, 2010). In addition to these existing projects, the Chinese government has committed more than US $70 million toward the construction of a second terminal at Abeid Amani Karume International Airport near Zanzibar City.

ANGOLA

Shifting over to the west coast of Africa, Angola has also benefitted from China's stadium diplomacy. Angola received four different football stadiums in 2009 in order for the state to host the 2010 Africa Cup of Nations (Coupe d'Afrique des Nations [CAN]; Caculo, 2009). These stadiums—Estádio 11 de Novembro, Estádio Nacional do Chiazi, Ombaka National Stadium, and Tundavala National Stadium—hosted much of the tournament and continue

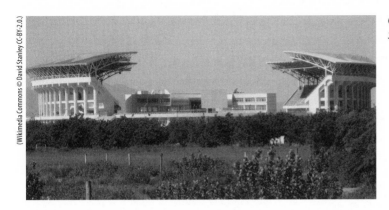

*Ombaka National
Stadium in Angola.*

to host matches today. Total costs were estimated to be about US $600 million (Will, 2012), which was financed by the Chinese government (Alm, 2012; Guest, 2009).

Estádio 11 de Novembro, the largest of the four stadiums, is located in Angola's capital city, Luanda. The stadium was named to honor Angola's Independence Day (Africa Ranking, 2015). The 50,000-seat stadium cost US $227 million and opened in 2009 (Alm, 2012). The stadium boasts two levels of seating, four VIP areas, 40 press boxes, two press rooms, accessible seating, and other modern amenities (Caculo, 2009). As the tournament's primary venue, Estádio 11 de Novembro hosted nine matches of the 2010 CAN, including five Group A, one Group B, one quarterfinal, one semifinal, and the final (World Public Library, 2015). Currently, the stadium is primarily used to host the Primerio de Agosto and Petro de Luanda football clubs as well as international matches (Buzz Nígería, 2015), but has been reported as showing signs of decline and deterioration (Will, 2012). Beyond hosting CAN, the construction of Estádio 11 de Novembro resonated with many local residents, who praised the addition of the stadium due to its effect on area development including infrastructure upgrades such as roads, piped water extensions, and electricity (Caculo, 2009).

Estádio Nacional do Chiazi, Ombaka National Stadium, and Tundavala National Stadium are noticeably smaller than Estádio 11 de Novembro but still held important roles in the 2010 CAN. Estádio Nacional do Chiazi, located in Cabinda, seats 20,000 including 204 VIP seats and 100 press seats. This stadium cost US $86 million (Alm, 2012). After hosting the 2010 CAN, FC de Cabinda made Estádio Nacional do Chiazi their home as the tenant team. With 35,000 seats, Ombaka National Stadium was the second largest stadium constructed for the 2010 CAN. Built with an unequal mix of Chinese and Angolan workers (BBC, 2009), Ombaka National Stadium cost US $118 million to build. Located in Benguela, it is now mostly used for football matches (Buzz Nígería, 2015). Finally, Tundavala National Stadium, located in Lubango, has a capacity of 20,000 and cost US $70 million (Alm, 2012).

JAMAICA

China's stadium diplomacy has also extended to the Caribbean. At the time of China's first venture there, the Caribbean was home to four of the 24 nation–states having diplomatic relations with Taiwan (discussed further in a later section). One example of China's stadium diplomacy in the Caribbean exists in Jamaica. Sligoville Stadium, named for the community in which it is located, is a multipurpose "mini-stadium" consisting of a 600-seat basketball and netball court, a 1,200-seat cricket oval, a 1,500-seat football pitch, and a 400-meter track (Brown, 2013). The Chinese government helped the Jamaican government design and construct the US $248-million complex after officials were approached by Jamaica's Minister of Foreign Affairs (Brown, 2013; Du, 2006). During the stadium's groundbreaking ceremony in 2006, China's Ambassador to Jamaica proclaimed that the facility was "not only a cooperative project between China and Jamaica, but also a good indication of the genuine friendship and sound relationship between the two countries" (Du, 2006, para. 5).

The venue was completed in 2007, but it went largely unutilized (Henry, 2013). A report from the *Jamaica Observer* described the stadium's deterioration:

> The chain-link fence enclosing the stadium is almost gone, having rotted away over the years. The plastic seats in the stands have crystallized, the majority of them completely destroyed. The bulbs and the casings for the floodlights on the court and the field are all broken. The goal nets are torn up, and the ankle-high grass acts as a deterrent even for those residents who might be inclined to hang out there. The gates, which were once locked to restrict unauthorized access, no longer serve that purpose as the fencing is also gone. While the facility still has electricity, there is no longer a caretaker to do regular landscaping of the venue. (Brown, 2013, para. 4)

The Chinese company that built the stadium expressed concern about its condition, leading them to question whether their resources were wasted on the development (Brown, 2013). In response, the Jamaican government recently planned to incorporate the Sligoville complex into the physical and programmatic structure at GC Foster College, a physical education and sport institute (Henry, 2013).

ANTIGUA AND BARBUDA

A second example of China's stadium diplomacy in the Caribbean exists in Antigua and Barbuda. The relationship between the two states stems from the 1980s, when Antigua and Barbuda became the first Caribbean nation–state to officially recognize China (Sheringham, 2007). The Chinese government built Sir Vivian Richards Stadium primarily for the 2007 Cricket World Cup hosted by Antigua and Barbuda. Sir Vivian Richards Stadium cost US $60 million and seats 10,000 fans (Williamson, 2015). The stadium was built after the Antiguan and Barbudan government contacted Beijing, who ultimately gifted Sir Vivian Richards Stadium to the state after a negotiation period (Embassy of the People's Republic of China in Antigua and Barbuda, 2011). After hosting the Cricket World Cup, the stadium continued to be used for cricket, with the Antigua and Barbuda and Leeward Islands cricket teams serving as the stadium's chief tenants (Williamson, 2015). The stadium has two main stands for spectators, a practice area, a new beach, training infrastructure, and a media center ("Sir Vivian Richards Stadium," 2007). Like other stadium projects supported by China, news accounts provided by the Chinese government and their diplomatic embassy have hailed Sir Vivian Richards Stadium for its contribution to the economic and infrastructural development of Antigua and Barbuda (e.g., Embassy of the People's Republic of China in Antigua and Barbuda, 2011).

COSTA RICA

Beyond the Caribbean, China's reach has also extended into Central America. Like the Caribbean, Central America is also an important area of diplomatic development for China, due in part to the number of states that provide diplomatic recognition of Taiwan (Will, 2012). Costa Rica and China forged a partnership with the construction of Estadio Nacional de Costa Rica (National Stadium), located in the capital city of San José. National Stadium opened in March 2011 and is Central America's first modern sport and event arena, replacing the old National Stadium, which was constructed in 1924 and torn down in 2008 (Williams, 2011a). The stadium seats 35,000 and has two jumbo screens including one 140-meter HD screen (Rodríguez, 2010), three decks of seating, office space, a sports museum, a hotel, and a banquet hall (Williams, 2011b). National Stadium is home to Costa Rica's national football team and also includes offices for 32 sport federations (Leandro, 2009). The stadium has hosted a number of concerts and major sporting events such as Pearl Jam, Shakira, Ricky Martin, Marc Anthony, the Jonas Brothers, Miley Cyrus, Megadeth, and friendly matches between Costa Rica's national team and Argentina, Brazil, and Spain (Williams, 2011b).

Cross-Strait instability was also an impetus to the development of National Stadium. In 2007, Costa Rica's then-President Óscar Arias severed ties with Taiwan in order to establish a partnership with China (Williams, 2011a). Next, San José Mayor Johnny Araya reached out directly to Beijing's mayor to request funding for National Stadium and to promote engagement between the two nation-states (Will, 2012). The Chinese government gifted the state "a token of appreciation" with the construction of a new National Stadium, spending about US$100 million on the project (Williams, 2011a, para. 5). Eight hundred Chinese workers were sent to Costa Rica to work shifts 24 hours a day in order to complete the project (Leandro, 2008).

Since National Stadium's opening, China has purchased patrol cars for the national police, provided credit for fixing up an oil refinery, bought US $300 million in bonds, and established a US $400 million loan for public transit and road construction. China also established a Confucius Institute in San José (Wilson, 2014). At the time National Stadium was being constructed, China's former ambassador to Costa Rica stated, "So far, Costa Rica hasn't given anything to China. But we are confident that in the future there will be projects that benefit both countries" (Robertson, 2009, para. 1). Two weeks after National Stadium opened, Costa Rica and China signed a free trade agreement (Davis, 2013). Additionally, with over 45,000 residents and a bustling Chinatown in the heart of San José, Costa Rica is now home to the second largest Chinese population in Central America (Will, 2012).

KIRIBATI

A clear illustration of the extent to which stadium diplomacy has been used as a political tool can be found in the Pacific island nation–state of Kiribati. There, China began construction of the Betio Sports Complex in 2002. This complex was the first national sporting center in Kiribati (Radio Australia, 2012). The US $5.5 million complex was expected to include basketball courts and a gymnasium capable of seating more than 1,000 spectators (Radio Australia, 2012). In return for the sports complex project, Kiribati cleared the Chinese government to build several satellite tracking stations designed to support China's space program (and, according to some defense analysts, spy on U.S. missile tests; Stratfor, 2003).

In 2003, however, the sports complex project was halted due to a shift in diplomatic relations between Kiribati and China. The change in status was spurred by the discovery that the Chinese ambassador to Kiribati donated money to an organization aligned with the current President Teburoro Tito, which created a major debate around the 2003 presidential election (Stratfor, 2003). Tito won reelection only to lose the presidency a year later after a vote of no confidence. The new president, Anote Tong, who was opposed to China's involvement, established diplomatic relations with Taiwan. In response, China dismantled its tracking stations and discontinued work on the sports complex, signaling its severing of diplomatic ties. The Betio Sports Complex was completed by the Taiwanese government and opened in 2006 (Marshall, 2007).

LAOS

As a final example of China's use of sports developments as a foreign policy strategy, China aided Laos in its endeavor to host the 25th Southeast Asian (SEA) Games in 2009. The New Laos National Stadium is a 20,000-seat facility located in Vientiane, the state's capital (McCartan, 2008). The stadium cost US $100 million and was financed by the China Development Bank (Stuart-Fox, 2009). In order to complete the project, thousands of Chinese workers were brought to Laos "due to the severe shortage of skilled Lao labor" (McCartan, 2008, para. 13). Three Chinese companies were contracted to construct the stadium; in exchange for the stadium, these companies were also given the rights to develop more than 4,000 acres of environmentally sensitive marshland for hotels and residences, shopping, and industry. The broad venture, coined the "New City Development Project," was portrayed as an anchor of the region's growing commercial enterprise (Stuart-Fox, 2009).

Despite China's significant investment in local infrastructure, Laotians expressed concern with the plan. First, locals feared that the New City Development Project's ownership would transform the development into a Chinatown, effectively crowding out Laotians both culturally and economically. Second, the proposed location for the development was in close proximity to Pha That Luang, an historic Buddhist site of national prominence (Stuart-Fox, 2009; Will, 2012). In response to these criticisms, Deputy Prime Minister Pomsavat Lengsavad defended the agreement with China, noting that the New Laos National Stadium and subsequent SEA Games would "showcase the country as a destination for investment and tourism" (McCartan, 2008, para. 5). Additionally, he attempted to assuage concerns about the New City Development Project by assuring Laotians that real estate would be open to all buyers, including the Lao and Chinese. Ultimately, the development in the That Luang marshes never materialized (Stuart-Fox, 2009).

These aforementioned examples illustrate China's investment in sports programs and infrastructure as a means of geopolitical strategy and international diplomacy. As discussed above, these partnerships were not without controversy, though the rationale for China's partnering with nation–states is relatively apparent. These cases exemplify how states (particularly those with emerging economies) may use sport as a vehicle to catalyze economic development or position themselves on the international stage (Kaplanidou, 2012). Indeed, many of the stadiums featured above were built specifically to host major sporting events such as the SEA Games, the CAN, or the Cricket World Cup. Below, we shift our attention to China's incentives for engaging in stadium diplomacy.

CHINA'S STAKE IN STADIUM DIPLOMACY

Despite Beijing's pronouncement that their grants and aid come without conditions, several examinations of China's foreign stadium projects have suggested that in addition to international diplomacy, Chinese investment has been driven by strategies aimed at growing its economy and strengthening its national defense. For instance, Rachel Will and Elliot Ross's separate reporting describes several different incentives for China's stadium diplomacy, including leverage in cross-Strait relations, access to valuable natural resources like oil, economic growth and entry into emerging markets, image-building before a worldwide audience, and the formation of strategic alliances that could prove useful when voting on United Nations resolutions (Ross, 2014; Will, 2011, 2012).

Cross-Strait influence is clearly an incentive for China's stadium diplomacy. In the above case studies, China–Taiwan diplomacy was an important consideration in Jamaica and Costa Rica. In Kiribati, the government's diplomatic shift from China to Taiwan resulted in a stadium complex started by the Chinese and completed by the Taiwanese. Today, there have been signs that cross-Strait relations may be improving, at least from the perspective of international trade and diplomatic cooperation. The 2008 announcement of a "diplomatic ceasefire" between China and Taiwan has put stadium diplomacy on hold in Latin America (Alexander, 2011; Wilson, 2014). While both sides are far from geopolitical harmony, they have respected the truce when it comes to sports developments. For example, when Taiwan-friendly Honduras considered establishing diplomatic relations with China in 2009, China "demurred in order to keep the peace" (Wilson, 2014, para. 9).

Like other nation–states competing in an international marketplace, China has established strategic partnerships in places rich with valuable resources or economic potential. For example, some oil-rich states, short on resources (both capital and human) to build infrastructure, can obtain loans in exchange for oil and gas rights. These states "pay steep interest rates and give up the rights to their natural resources for years. China has a lock on close to 90 percent of Ecuador's oil exports, which mostly goes to paying off its loans" (Krauss & Bradsher, 2015, p. 1A).

Other economic incentives include the ability to employ Chinese workers on the projects. The large number of laborers utilized for mega projects often necessitates additional development (e.g., residences, shopping centers, dining) to accommodate the influx of foreign nationals, an example of which was the New City Development Project in Laos. For China, these developments can be economically rewarding, but they can also spur controversy. For example, in Angola, China's leading oil supplier (Chadwick, 2015), more than 40,000 Chinese laborers were used for comprehensive post-war reconstruction; this group represented nearly 90% of the total construction workforce ("Angolan Gangs," 2009). Chinese companies were awarded several key contracts on projects that included roads, airports, government buildings, and the four stadiums used for the 2010 CAN. Tension from the influx of Chinese workers in Angola eventually erupted into violence when Angolan gangs began targeting Chinese companies and workers. Reports of violence against Chinese workers included murders, robberies by gunpoint, beatings, and torture (Obajo Ori, 2009). Despite the pushback, China's partnership with Angola has been called a game-changer; by 2010, Angola was China's largest African trade partner (Power, Mohan, & Tan-Mullins, 2012).

Finally, stadium diplomacy may uniquely help the sponsoring state construct a public image that showcases the goodwill of its humanitarian efforts and the legitimacy of its government. Stadiums and international competitions may uniquely contribute to this branding, given the large audiences often associated with sporting events. Much like China has done by hosting its own major events over the past 10 years (i.e., 2008 Summer Olympic and Paralympic Games, 2010 World Expo, and 2010 Asian Games), its participation in the highly publicized opening of an ally's national stadium can enhance its image among the host state, the Chinese, and a worldwide audience (Chen, 2012). On the other hand, stadium developments embroiled in controversy may affect both the recipient state and China. For example, similar to the challenges of any urban stadium project, Costa Rica's National Stadium and Antigua's Sir Vivian Richards Stadium have both been criticized for their locations, reflecting the idea that the facilities were poorly planned and hastily constructed. Commenting on National Stadium, former Culture Minister Guido Sáenz called the stadium's location in San José's city center "a catastrophe" (Williams, 2011a, para. 15). Sir Vivian Richards Stadium has been dogged by low attendance, blamed on the facility's distance from the Antiguan and Barbudan capital of St. John's (Williamson, 2015). Finally, China has been criticized for its failure to help maintain its stadium developments post-opening. Similar to the state of Jamaica's Sligoville Stadium, Angola's four CAN stadiums, all still in their infancy, have "slid into a permanent decline" (Will, 2012, p. 43). These problems reinforce the view that China's stadium diplomacy is less about forging local legacies in recipient states and more about its positioning as a world power.

CONCLUSION

China's rise as an economic power may trouble its rivals, not only due to China's influence on international trade and policy, but also because of the harmful effects it could have on the global economy:

> The show of financial strength also makes China—and the world—more vulnerable. Long an engine of global growth, China is taking on new risks by exposing itself to shaky political regimes, volatile emerging markets and other economic forces beyond its control. (Krauss & Bradsher, 2015, p. 1A)

Looking ahead, China's robust investments abroad are expected to continue. With an estimated US $4 trillion in foreign currency reserves, there is little evidence to suggest it will reduce its foreign aid spending (Krauss & Bradsher, 2015). While China's stadium developments have slowed in some regions, they continued to be active throughout Africa. Cape Verde's Estádio Nacional opened in 2014 (backed by a US $12-million, 20-year loan), while Malawi's 40,000-seat, US $70-million Bingu National Stadium was completed in 2015 (Escobar & Simões, 2013; Khamula, 2015). China is also building stadiums in Gabon and Ivory Coast for the 2017 and 2021 CAN, respectively (Kazeem, 2015).

Just as China's stadium diplomacy is unlikely to subside, it is unlikely to be adopted as a tool of geopolitical strategy elsewhere. In the past several years, citizens in several democratic states have shown strong opposition to financing sports projects in their own homelands. The recent defeat of multiple Olympic-bid referendums in European cities prompted several mainstream media reporters to question whether mega-events like the World Cup and Olympic and Paralympic Games would ever be held in a democratic state after Brazil (Applebaum, 2014; Chandler, 2014). It is also likely that many nation–states would reject the offer of a sponsoring government to finance a stadium development. In South America, for example, there would be little enthusiasm for an offer of stadium diplomacy. Wilson (2014) explains:

> With the notable exception of Paraguay, every country recognizes [China], and all have a tendency to have a nationalistic relationship to sport. Having a foreign country finance a stadium might wound national pride, and wouldn't necessarily change their economic or political fortunes. As it stands, they can pursue trade and investment without the appearance of a bribe, and keep their political and cultural integrity intact. (para. 10)

Of course, it is also worth noting that few economies have the capacity to invest in outward development as heavily as China.

Though a small part of its overall foreign aid spending, China's stadium diplomacy has been an effective geopolitical tool. Increasing influence in cross-Strait relations, the acquisition of valuable oil rights, the forming of strategic partnerships around the world, and an enhanced public image have all occurred under China's foreign stadium developments. Premised on the expectation that a major sports stadium and the events held within it will stimulate a developing state's economy, governments throughout Africa, the Caribbean, Central America, and the South Pacific have partnered with China to construct sports infrastructure. Critics of these diplomatic unions (some of whom include the recipient state's own citizens) are distrustful of Beijing's portrayal of stadium aid as unconditional, instead claiming the recipient is being exploited for resources, political gain, or economic improvement. All signs suggest that China's already sizable stadium diplomacy program will continue to grow. As demonstrated here, scholars, analysts, and ordinary citizens have characterized this program in contrasting or even contradictory ways: as creating opportunity and as opportunistic, as coming with no strings attached or as based on a quid pro quo, as working toward a cross-Strait truce or as a strategic move toward One China. The continued observation of developments in this area may be the only way to settle these analytic disputes.

DISCUSSION QUESTIONS

1. What examples of other nation–states' foreign aid parallel China's stadium diplomacy?

2. In your view, what motives underlie China's comprehensive foreign aid programs?

3. Should nation–states like the United States or Australia adopt programs similar to China's stadium diplomacy? Why or why not?

4. In your opinion, why do you think China's stadium diplomacy has been successful?

5. How does China's stadium diplomacy reflect on the nature of sports around the world?

REFERENCES

Africa Ranking. (2015). Top 10 most expensive stadiums in Africa. Retrieved from http://www.africaranking.com/most-expensive-stadiums-in-africa/3/

Alexander, C. (2011). Public diplomacy and the diplomatic truce: Taiwan and the People's Republic of China (PRC) in El Salvador. *Place Branding and Public Diplomacy, 7,* 271–288.

Alm, J. (2012). *World stadium index.* Copenhagen, Denmark: Danish Institute for Sports Studies/Play the Game.

Angolan Gangs Go After Chinese. (2009, November 13). *News24.* Retrieved from http://www.news24.com/Africa/News/Angolan-gangs-go-after-Chinese-20091113

Applebaum, A. (2014, June 12). Democracy's last World Cup? *Slate.* Retrieved from http://www.slate.com

BBC. (2009). Inside Angola's 2010 stadiums. Retrieved from http://news.bbc.co.uk/sport2/hi/football/africa/8253430.stm

Bernal, R. L. (2015). The growing economic presence of China in the Caribbean. *The World Economy, 38,* 1409–1437.

Bräutigam, D. (2011). Aid 'with Chinese characteristics': Chinese foreign aid and development finance meet the OECD-DAC aid regime. *Journal of International Development, 23,* 752–764.

Brown, I. (2013, May 19). Chinese lament waste of money on Sligoville mini-stadium. *Jamaica Observer.* Retrieved from http://www.jamaicaobserver.com/news/Stadium-built-with-Chinese-money-in-ruins_14278481

Buzz Nígería. (2015). 10 African stadiums that cost a fortune to construct... You won't believe where number 1 is located. Retrieved from http://buzznigeria.com/10-african-stadiums-that-cost-a-fortune-to-construct-you-wont-believe-where-number-1-is-located/

Caculo, P. (2009, December 27). Estádio 11 de Novembro Stadium is inaugurated today. *Journal dos Desportos.* Retrieved from http://jornaldosdesportos.sapo.ao/24/0/estadio_11_de_novembro_e_hoje_inagurado

Chadwick, S. (2015, June 24). Why Africa excels at sport, but not the sport industry. *Business Day Live.* Retrieved from http://www.bdlive.co.za/opinion/2015/06/24/why-africa-excels-at-sport-but-not-the-sport-industry

Chandler, A. (2014, October 1). What if democracies refuse to pay for the Olympics again? *The Atlantic.* Retrieved from http://www.theatlantic.com

Chen, N. (2012). Branding national images: The 2008 Beijing Summer Olympics, 2010 Shanghai World Expo, and 2010 Guangzhou Asian Games. *Public Relations Review, 38,* 731–745.

Davis, N. (2013, September 4). How a Chinese-funded Costa Rican soccer stadium explains the world. *Pacific Standard.* Retrieved from http://www.psmag.com/business-economics/chinese-funded-costa-rican-soccer-stadium-explains-world-65667

Du, J. (2006, March 24). China helps Jamaica build sports complex. State Council of the People's Republic of China. Retrieved from http://www.gov.cn/misc/2006-03/24/content_235586.htm

Embassy of the People's Republic of China in Antigua and Barbuda. (2011). H. E. Mr. Lui Hanming, Ambassador of the People's Republic of China to Antigua and Barbuda, receives exclusive interview by the ABS TV of Antigua and Barbuda. Retrieved from http://ag.china-embassy.org/eng/xwfw/t865469.htm

Embassy of the People's Republican of China in the United Republic of Tanzania. (2010, May 21). Speech by Ambassador Liu Xinsheng on the handing-over ceremony of the rehabilitation project of Zanzibar Amaan Stadium. Retrieved from http://tz.china-embassy.org/eng/xwdt/t696087.htm

Escobar, A., & Simões, J. K. (2013, December 13). Building on ambition–China helps build Cape Verde after independence. *Macauhub.* Retrieved from http://www.macauhub.com.mo/en/2013/12/13/building-on-ambition-china-helps-build-cape-verde-after-independence/

Grimm, S. (2011). Transparency of Chinese aid: An analysis of the published information on Chinese external financial flows. *Publish what you fund—Centre for Chinese Studies.* Retrieved from http://www.aidtransparency.net/wp-content/uploads/2011/08/Transparency-of-Chinese-Aid_final.pdf

Guest, A. (2009, November 16). Building stadiums: Angola, China, and the African Cup of Nations. Pitch invasion. Retrieved from http://www.pitchinvasion.com

Henry, B. (2013). Ruined Sligoville Stadium to be rescued, says Neita-Headley. *Jamaica Observer.* Retrieved from http://www.jamaicaobserver.com/news/Ruined-Sligoville-Stadium-to-be-rescued--says-Neita-Headley_14435373

Information Office of the State Council. (2011). China's foreign aid [White paper]. Retrieved from http://www.gov.cn/english/official/2011-04/21/content_1849913.htm

Information Office of the State Council. (2014). China's foreign aid [White paper]. Retrieved from http://english.gov.cn/archive/white_paper/2014/08/23/content_281474982986592.htm

International Monetary Fund. (2014). *External debt statistics: Guide for compilers and users.* Washington, DC: International Monetary Fund.

Juma, M. (2013, December 17). Tanzania: Rain delays Amaan Stadium artificial turf. Retrieved from http://allafrica.com/stories/201312170152.html

Kaplanidou, K. (2012). The importance of legacy outcomes for Olympic Games four summer host cities' quality of life: 1996–2008. *European Sport Management Quarterly, 12,* 397–433.

Kazeem, Y. (2015, July 15). How China will play a key role as Gabon hosts 2017 AFCON. *Ventures Africa.* Retrieved from http://venturesafrica.com/how-china-will-play-a-key-role-as-gabon-hosts-2017-afcon/

Kellison, T. B., & Mondello, M. J. (2012). Organisational perception management in sport: The use of corporate pro-environmental behaviour for desired facility referenda outcomes. *Sport Management Review, 15,* 500–512. doi:10.1016/j.smr.2012.01.005

Khamula, O. (2015, December 3). Malawi govt delays China-funded Bingu stadium handover. *Nyasa Times.* Retrieved from http://www.nyasatimes.com/2015/12/03/malawi-govt-delays-china-funded-bingu-stadium-handover/

Krauss, C., & Bradsher, K. (2015, July 26). China's global ambitions, cash and strings attached. *The New York Times,* p. 1A.

Kudos to Karume for Refurbishing Stadium. (2010, May 22). *Guardian.* Retrieved from http://www.ippmedia.com/frontend/?l=16957

Leandro, H. (2008, May 13). Comenzó demolición del Estadio Nacional. *La Nación.* Retrieved from http://wvw.nacion.com/ln_ee/2008/mayo/13/deportes1534115.html

Leandro, H. (2009, July 28). Levantan la primera gradería del Nuevo Estadio Nacional. *La Nación.* Retrieved from http://wvw.nacion.com/ln_ee/2009/julio/28/deportes2040316.html

Marshall, I. (2007, September 24). Kiribati rises to the occasion to host outstanding development visit. Retrieved from http://www.ittf.com/stories/Stories_detail.asp?ID=13482&Category=&General_Catigory=Development%2C+general%2C+Waiting&

McCartan, B. (2008, July 26). New-age Chinatown has Laotians on edge. *Asia Times.* Retrieved from http://www.atimes.com/atimes/Southeast_Asia/JG26Ae02.html

Obajo Ori, K. (2009, November 14). Angola: Chinese violence and murders, protest or criminality? *Afrik News.* Retrieved from http://www.afrik-news.com/article16469.html

Office of the Historian. (2015). The Chinese revolution of 1949. U.S. Department of State. Retrieved from https://history.state.gov/milestones/1945-1952/chinese-rev

Power, M., Mohan, G., & Tan-Mullins, M. (2012). *China's resource diplomacy in Africa: Powering development?* Houndmills, UK: Palgrave Macmillan.

Radio Australia. (2012, March 26). Foundations laid for Kiribati sports complex. Retrieved from http://www.radioaustralia.net.au/international/2002-11-28/foundations-laid-for-kiribati-sports-complex/601424

Robertson, M. (2009, March 20). Stadium construction begins, crisis or not. *Tico Times.* Retrieved from http://www.ticotimes.net/2009/03/20/stadium-construction-begins-crisis-or-not

Rodríguez, J. L. (2010, August 24). Estadio Nacional tendrá pantalla de 140 metros HD. Retrieved from http://www.nacion.com/deportes/otros-deportes/Estadio-Nacional-pantalla-metros-HD_0_1142685745.html

Ross, E. (2014, January 28). China's stadium diplomacy in Africa. *Roads & Kingdoms.* Retrieved from http://www.roadsandkingdoms.com

Sheringham, S. (2007, March 7). China splurges on Caribbean cricket in quest to isolate Taiwan. *Bloomberg.* Retrieved from http://www.bloomberg.com/apps/news?pid=newsarchive&sid=ajv47UQW6sq8

Sir Vivian Richards Stadium, North Sound, Antigua. (2007, February 27). That's cricket. Retrieved from http://www.thatscricket.com/news/2007/02/27/2702sir-vivian-richards-stadium-antigua.html

SMZ to Protect Amaan Stadium. (2010, April 1). *Guardian.* Retrieved from http://www.ippmedia.com/frontend/index.php?l=15113

Stratfor. (2003, November 7). Kiribati and diplomatic relations: Whither China's space program? Retrieved from https://www.stratfor.com/analysis/kiribati-and-diplomatic-relations-whither-chinas-space-program

Stuart-Fox, M. (2009). Laos: The Chinese connection. In D. Singh (Ed.), *Southeast Asian Affairs 2009.* (pp. 141–169). Singapore: Institute of Southeast Asian Studies.

Wang, B., Mao, R., & Gou, Q. (2014). Overseas impacts of China's outward direct investment. *Asian Economic Policy Review, 9,* 227–249.

Will, R. (2011, November 21). China's stadium diplomacy. *US-China Today.* Retrieved from http://www.uschina.usc.edu/article@usct?chinas_stadium_diplomacy_17566.aspx

Will, R. (2012). China's stadium diplomacy. *World Policy Journal, 29*(2), 36–43.

Williams, A. (2011a, March 24). Costa Rica's 35,000-seat National Stadium opens. *Tico Times.* Retrieved from http://www.ticotimes.net/2011/03/25costa-rica-s-35-000-seat-national-stadium-opens

Williams, A. (2011b, December 21). Big stars, great shows at National Stadium. *Tico Times.* Retrieved from http://wvw.nacion.com/ln_ee/2008/mayo/13/deportes1534115.html

Williamson, M. (2015). Sir Vivian Richards Stadium. Retrieved from http://www.espncricinfo.com/westindies/content/ground/208543.html

Wilson, T. (2014, August 26). Latin America and the twilight of China's stadium diplomacy. *Nearshore Americas.* Retrieved from http://www.nearshoreamericas.com/latin-america-twilight-chinas-stadium-diplomacy/

World Public Library. (2015). Estádio 11 de Novembro. Retrieved from http://self.gutenberg.org/articles/Est%C3%A1dio_11_de_Novembro

9

WRESTLING WITH DIPLOMACY: THE UNITED STATES AND IRAN

SOOLMAZ ABOOALI

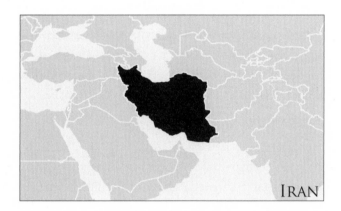

IRAN

INTRODUCTION: STATE OF AFFAIRS

Part I

I am an Iranian-American, and I am an athlete. I am also a refugee who left my homeland at an early age to later settle in the land that I now call home—the United States. You can imagine my excitement when, in 1998, I traveled to Stade Gerland stadium in Lyon, France, to watch the Iranian and American soccer teams "duke it out" on the field in what was the FIFA World Cup. Little did I know that I was about to witness the power of sport collide with the power of politics. Halfway through the match, the stadium turned white and yellow as spectators donned t-shirts and waved banners in support for the largest opposition organization against the Iranian government. The game was halted for a short while, the crowd continued to wear their white-yellow colors, and the message that political opposition was alive and well was waved in the world's face.

As a child, this moment was etched in my mind, a moment I knew I had to understand more deeply. I wondered how the athletes had felt during the pause, and I wondered also what results, if any, the political demonstration would produce for relations between Iran and the United States. American philanthropist Ted Turner coined the phrase "sport is war without the killing," and this may hold a kernel of truth in the usual zero-sum nature of sporting events and the emotions sport can invoke among spectators. My first-hand experiences as an athlete have demonstrated the opposite: it is exactly within these moments of chaos and competition that ripe opportunities are also presented to humanize the "others."

International martial arts competition has taught me that two opposing fighters can engage in intense, heated conflict and still remain comrades before and after the actual bout. The human ability to move from a me-versus-the-other perspective to one of 'we' is not weakened by these conflicts; rather, it can become stronger through a common bond.

The question is—can sporting events provide soft power opportunities wherein athletes, who hold a certain platform of influence within their respective societies, foster understanding through engagement beyond the moment and toward furthering diplomatic aims? We explore this question through an examination of Iranian–American conflicts, sport exchanges, and how this type of interaction can influence relations.

Part II: Iran and United States—Frenemies

In 2015, the Joint Comprehensive Plan of Action (JCPOA) agreement between the United States and the Islamic Republic captured the world's attention. After two years of direct negotiations, Iran agreed to reduce its stockpile of medium-enriched uranium by 98% and idle roughly two-thirds of its active centrifuges for at least 15 years. While Iran can continue to enrich uranium to 3.67%, it will restrict this activity to a single facility for 10 years. In return for Iran's submission to these constraints, the United States, European Union, and United Nations Security Council agreed to lift economic and diplomatic sanctions against the Islamic Republic (Samore, 2015). This agreement is the latest landmark in an on-again, off-again relationship between the United States and Iran that has spanned decades. After the United Kingdom and the Soviet Union invaded Iran during World War II, the US became closely engaged with postwar recovery and detente. The United States and its postwar allies (notably the United Kingdom) had a strong economic interest in Iranian oil, pressuring the Iranian government to agree to contracts favorable to those countries. (Byrne, 2015).

Relations took a sharp dip in the early 1950s when Iran's Prime Minister, Mohammed Mosaddegh, requested an audit of the Anglo-Iranian Oil Company (AIOC), a British corporation (now BP) that was engaged in the export of Iranian oil. According to Iranian testimonials, Mosaddegh was wary of the confrontation that this request could provoke but was himself under considerable pressure from Iran's religious community (Kressin, 1991).

When AIOC rejected Iran's request, Iran's parliament (the Majlis) nationalized the company's assets and expelled its representatives from the country. The US and UK responded sharply, engendering a coup against Mosaddegh (called Operation AJAX) and placing Iran in the hands of Shah Mohammad-Reza Pahlavi. In subsequent decades, Pahlavi became

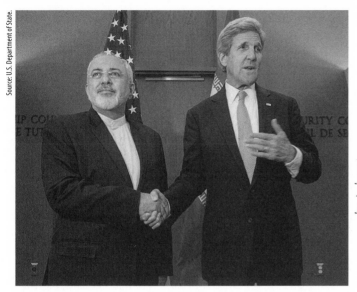

Source: U.S. Department of State.

U.S. Secretary of State John Kerry and Iranian Ambassador Mohammad Javad Zarif

increasingly dependent upon Western support to maintain his monarchy (Byrne & Gasi-orowski, 2004). Pahlavi's close relationship with the US and the secular nature of his rule engendered resentment and distrust among Iran's religious community, which participated in strikes and demonstrations against his rule in 1977 and 1978 (Abrahamian, 1982). The Shah chose exile in 1979 and was granted asylum in the United States (Daugherty, 2003).

The revolutionary movement welcomed Ayatollah Ruhollah Khomeini back from exile in France and gave him the office of Supreme Leader (Abrahamian, 1982). On April 1, 1979, Iran declared itself to be an Islamic Republic (Abrahamian 1982). The United States' continued support of Pahlavi prompted the new Iranian government to allow the occupation of the American embassy in Tehran, triggering a 444-day long hostage crisis during which 52 American diplomats were held in Tehran (Farber, 2005).

After the kidnapping, the United States severed all relations with Iran, freezing $12 B of the country's foreign assets (Brower & Brueschke, 1998). In 1995, President Bill Clinton imposed further economic sanctions, which were renewed by the Bush administration (Clawson, 2010). Iran's pursuit of a uranium enrichment program—and its implications for Iran's development of a nuclear arsenal—prompted international escalation of sanctions and repeated inspections of its enrichment facilities by the International Atomic Energy Administration (Cordesman & Al-Rodhan, 2006).

Throughout this time, the two countries engaged in mutual provocation and directed rhetoric, such as President Bush's inclusion of Iran in his "Axis of Evil" (Segell, 2005, p. 153), American support of expatriate Iranian resistance groups such as the Mujaheddin al-Khalq (MEK; USG, 2006), the arrest and trial of Iranian-American dual citizens by the Islamic Republic on charges of espionage (Morello, 2015), and incursion into Iranian territory by United States drones (Tyson, 2005). The discussions that led to the JCPOA represented the first direct negotiations between the two countries in over thirty years.

While negotiations have proven to be fraught with contention, one item that Iranians and Americans alike can agree upon is their passion for sport. Indeed, sport has become a cultural fixture in both countries.

SPORT AS A COMMON CULTURE

Iran's affinity for sport has been present throughout its history, its location and geography reflecting its athletic tradition. From polo to wrestling to football (soccer), Iranians enjoy sport both as a pastime and as a competitive endeavor. One fundamental representative institution is the *zoorkhaneh* ("House of Strength"), a gymnasium of sorts that represents an indigenous athletic tradition (Chehabi, 2002, p. 276; Kiani & Faraji, 2011). The zoorkhaneh was traditionally a place that prepared athletes for wrestling, until international freestyle and Greco-Roman wrestling replaced the previously established wrestling styles of the zoorkhaneh.

Exercises in the zoorkhaneh are accompanied by chanted verses from Iran's national epic the Shahnameh (*Book of Kings,* an epic poem dated from 1000 AD). The zoorkhanehs are thus tightly coupled with Iranian history and culture, "meaning that this traditional institution could be harnessed for the ideological purposes of the state, which promoted Iranian nationalism" (Chehabi, 2002, p. 280). The exercises also mimic the martial arts of the Persian soldiers of the Sassanid era, turning war into sport to increase national pride (Zakeri, 1995).

A leading zoorkhaneh practitioner, Sha'ban Ja'fari, was instrumental in the CIA-backed coup d'état that ousted Prime Minister Mohammad Mossadegh and leader of the National Front that insisted on governing Iran without the Shah's and Western (British and US) influence (Chehabi, 2002; Rahnema, 2015; Limbert, 2009). For this service he was decorated, appointed as the head of the traditional athletics establishment, and supported to build his own athletic club called the Ja'fari Club (Rahnema, 2015).

Another well-known Iranian sports figure is Gholamreza Takhti (Chehabi, 1995). In 1962, an earthquake shattered the city of Buin Zahra in western Iran, killing 45,000 people. Takhti, also known by Iranians as Jahān Pahlevān or The World Champion, took matters into his own hands and decided to provide assistance. Takhti was an Olympic gold medalist and world champion wrestler known not only for his skills on the mat but also for his chivalrous, socially conscious character as both an athlete and citizen.

Shortly following the earthquake, Takhti walked the streets of Tehran to knock on doors and ask for financial assistance for those affected by the natural disaster. It was said that he carried around a large bucket that was filled with monetary donations by the end of his house rounds. Through such efforts, Takhti mobilized the public to provide for basic human needs and mitigate the effects of the conflict on the well-being of those touched by it.

Takhti also supported the National Front but continued to enjoy popular acclaim across all sectors of society and political spectrum. At an international match, for example, Takhti refused to wrestle in order to stand in solidarity with other top wrestlers who had grievances with the lack of social security provided by the Shah's regime. Spectators chanted Takhti's name and refused to let the games begin until he allowed them to; Takhti had gained more leverage than government officials and the royal family, including the Shah's brother, who was present at the game and witnessed such influence (Chehabi, 2002).

Takhti and Ja'fari provide examples of Iranian athletes practicing culturally significant sports who accrued the mass-power to dampen or alter the influence of political figures in some shape or form. Iranian athletics are not restricted to traditional sports, of course. As a result of British colonialism and participation in international competitions, Iranians became quite enamored with other sports such as football, softball, and volleyball (Guttman 2007), with the men's volleyball team ranked number one in Asia in 2015. The adoption and inclusion of these Western games and their enshrinement alongside traditional sports are examples of culture supporting, encouraging, and creating meaning around the importance of sport in Iranian society. Culture is indeed a significant factor, as it is the "derivative of experience...deeply connected to ongoing or past social practice" (Avruch, 2013, p. 11).

Sport has tremendous influence in the United States as well. We have seen the rise of organized sports and free-play in schools, in parks and recreation centers, and a general national push for more active citizens (Aspen Institute, 2015; PSCFN, 2015). While baseball is the national sport of the country (Block, 2005; Morris, 2006), basketball and soccer have also enjoyed national growth in participation and spectatorship. The US also demonstrates connections between sports, politics, and ideology in many forms, including beginning each sporting event with the singing of the national anthem. President Nixon, appropriately code-named "Quarterback" by the Secret Service, began the tradition of making congratulatory calls to players after victorious championships (Billings, Butterworth, & Turman, 2015); U.S. presidents throw ceremonial first pitches at baseball games, a symbolic tradition first started by President Howard Taft in 1910 and carried out by each president thereafter. The US boycotted the 1980 Summer Olympics in Moscow, a decision motivated by opposition to Russia's invasion of Afghanistan.

In America, sport is a cultural institution and generates a sense of community. When politicians involve themselves in the world, they are attempting to relate to others and demonstrate that they are in touch with American culture, using sport metaphors such as "bring it home," "a new ball game," and "drop the ball," among others. For example, U.S. presidents invite seven sports teams to the White House each year to celebrate their achievements, ones "they claim support their vision and national unity and American values" (Billings et al., 2015, pp. 167-68).

Sport has also played a significant role in the political arena. Babe Ruth's positive reputation as an ambassador of baseball through his many visits to Japan was used by the US as a means to promote its foreign policy. Before World War I, both the U.S. and Major League Baseball believed hostilities with Japan could be avoided through the sport loved by both nations. Later, it was used to communicate aggression, and during World War II, Japanese soldiers invoked Babe Ruth to insult American soldiers, yelling phrases such as "To hell with Babe Ruth!" or "Fuck Babe Ruth!" (Elias, 2011).

Later in the war, Babe Ruth's influence was once again invoked. The State Department proposed that he make a radio announcement urging the Japanese to surrender before the bombing of Hiroshima and Nagasaki (Elias, 2011). During the reconstruction of Japan after World War II, other popular baseball players, including Lefty O'Doul, were called upon in hope that their popularity would help occupying forces to boost morale and prevent the spread of communism.

Baseball was also leveraged to play a role in post-WWII America, a time when African Americans were seeking equality in the US. Professional sports, notably baseball, became one venue in which equality was demonstrated (Hill, 2007). Jackie Robinson effectively showed his ability to play ball side by side with white players without being deterred by the tremendous backlash he received from teammates, fans, and the media. The dialogue and awareness of Jackie Robinson's presence shined the spotlight on deeply ingrained racial barriers in the country at that time. Indeed, baseball has been known to tell the

> story of race in America . . . of immigration and assimilation. . . . [T]he game
> is a repository of age-old American verities, of standards against which we
> continually measure ourselves, and yet at the same time a mirror of the pres-
> ent moment in our modern culture. (Reiss, 1999, p. xiii)

Other athletes have also propelled social change throughout American history. In 1967, boxer Muhammad Ali stood behind his political and religious beliefs in the face of incarceration; in the 1970s, tennis player Billie Jean King's social and political impact paved the way for gender equity rights, particularly as they related to equal pay. And we would remiss if we did not mention the show of kindness, the small gift given in 1971 by Chinese table tennis player Zhuang Zedong to American Glenn Cowan that, once captured by media, played a role in helping to spur discussions between Chinese and U.S. state actors.

Sport in such examples has been used as a means to promote culture and a set of ideas, a means to create and perpetuate specific results that benefit the nation. To better understand how nations have traditionally undertaken approaches to advance their goals, we turn the discussion to diplomacy.

THE CHANGING FACE OF DIPLOMACY

Since the mid-seventeenth century, diplomacy has been both institution and mechanism for international affairs (Murray, 2012). Traditional diplomacy was defined as the "conduct of relations between sovereign states with standing in world politics by official agents and by peaceful means" (Bull, 1977, p. 156). The oft-misquoted Prussian general von Clausewitz recognized diplomacy as a tool with many mechanisms at its disposal, including war. His aphorism that war is "not merely a political act, but also a real political instrument, a continuation of policy, a carrying out of the same by other means" (von Clausewitz, 1918, p. 23) introduced the perspective that war is an element of diplomacy, not its absence). In other words, diplomacy does not cease to exist in the absence of diplomats—it continues during open conflict.

Traditional diplomacy's inability to quickly adapt to the changing geopolitical structures has created a vacuum, an opportunity seized by nongovernmental and international organizations, philanthropic figures, and athletes who have begun to act as nonstate diplomatic actors affecting international relations. In their attempts to evolve, foreign affairs ministries have attempted to learn from the corporate sector, where people are identified as the "only real resource in diplomacy" (Murray, 2012, p. 7).

As a contrast to hard power's *push* focus, meaning that it imposes its perspective by force, Joseph Nye asks us to consider the addition of *soft power,* which is "the enormous capacity of this country to get what it wants by attraction rather than through coercion." (Nye, 2006, p. 85). Soft power therefore *pulls,* using attraction. Another aspect of soft power is *engagement,* specifically cultivating and maintaining relationships with citizens and influencers within another country.

The use of sport as a medium of cultural exchange is a form of soft power. Politics in today's era has become a contest of competitive credibility (Nye, 2008). The world of traditional power politics is typically scored via military or economic victories, the idea of nations using material resources to influence or compel other nations. Politics in an information age "may ultimately be about whose story wins" (Arquila and Ronfeldt, 1999, p. 53)—for example, stories can be emitted through cultural exchanges that utilize sport. The rise of technologies has undoubtedly led to easier, faster, and cheaper transmission of vast amounts of information which is "transforming how people think, organize, and connect" (Gregory, 2014, p. 8). With such an "abundance of information" (Simon, 1998, p. 30) to sift through and absorb, people tend to lose attention and focus. As scholar Herbert Simon states, "a wealth of knowledge creates a poverty of attention" (Simon, 1971, p. 40). Those who are able to guide periods of attention and focus possess the power to influence the masses, and among those who attempt to do so credibility becomes something to compete for and an important facet of soft power (Nye, 2008, p. 100). Scholar Joseph Nye (2003) places soft power as the third pillar of policy for the US, alongside military and economic power. This is necessary, he asserts, because even a country as strong as the US cannot rely solely upon unilateral action (emblematic of hard power) to achieve its diplomatic goals. Multilateralism is thus not optional—it is necessary in light of the fall of the Soviet Union and the consequent inability of the two great powers to ignore the United Nations (Aviel, 2005). The United States and other powers must invest significantly more money for aid, information, educational, cultural, and other programs in order for this framework to succeed. Nye regards the diplomatic world as a "complex arena in which a nation's purposes are pursued through constant interaction with others. You change them and they change you in a never-ending process" (Woollacott, 2002, par. 9). Perhaps it is the adoption of this perspective that has moved the US away from unilateral, hard power actions in its relationship with Iran (such as the coup against Mosaddegh) toward the P5+1 talks that produced the recent nuclear accord.

Twenty years ago, Australian politician Gareth Evans defined public diplomacy as "an exercise in persuasion and influence that extends beyond traditional diplomacy by leveraging a much larger cast of players both inside and outside government" (Evans & Grant, 1995, p. 66). For example, Rome's *vox populi* (Latin for "voice of the people") phenomenon now spans the globe. Social media—a tool that was inconceivable during von Clausewitz's era—is now a tool of modern statecraft, both traditional and public. Social media has altered the ways in which governments and people interact, as well as how a "nation sets up its diplomatic strategies and actuates its foreign policy agenda and objectives" (Sandre, 2013, p. 9). The basic distinction between traditional and public diplomacy is straightforward: the former is about relationships between the representatives of states or other international actors, whereas the latter targets the general public in foreign societies and more specific nonofficial groups, organizations, and individuals.

The United States Department of State's Office of Public Diplomacy and Public Affairs recognizes this distinction, using public diplomacy to

> support the achievement of U.S. foreign policy goals and objectives, advance national interests, and enhance national security by informing and influencing foreign publics and by expanding and strengthening the relationship between the people and Government of the United States and citizens of the rest of the world. (USDS, n.d., par. 1)

Soft power falls under this umbrella. In conjunction with public diplomacy, it has been extremely effective as a tool to both disseminate national perspectives and make them appealing. Saudi Arabia, for example, has spent millions across decades on schools, mosques, and informational campaigns to promote Wahhabism, an interpretation of Islam woven deeply into its government and thus its goals and policies (Choksy & Choksy 2015).

As a more focused example, Grand Ayatollah Ruhollah Khomeini created an organization that relied upon thousands of students to distribute cassette tapes of his sermons and speeches in mosques, universities, and streets across Iran (Brumberg, 2001). These messages exhorted Iranians to revolt against US-backed Shah Reza Pahlavi, equating him with Yazid, a historical usurper of Islamic power. It was therefore, according to Khomeini, their religious duty to defeat the Shah and usher in the return of Shia Islam's Twelfth Imam (Dabashi, 2008). Once the people overthrew the government, Khomeini returned to Iran and claimed the title of Supreme Leader, demonstrating the effectiveness of soft power and public diplomacy.

The combination of religion, soft power, and public diplomacy is not limited to Islam. Pope Francis, head of the Catholic Church, has demonstrated both understanding and skill in Nye's soft power (Ignatius, 2015). He relies upon speeches, appearances, publications, and social media to further the Church's goals and spread its message to the populace. Centuries removed from its history of hard power, the Vatican has adroitly taken up the reins of public diplomacy and soft power in pursuit of its goals.

Surprisingly, athletes have become agents of soft power and public diplomacy as well. For example, SportsUnited is a division within the United States Department of State that invites teams of athletes from around the world into the country to engage with other sports-minded individuals and teams as a means to promote mutual understanding and "transcend linguistic and sociocultural differences" (USDS, BECA, 2016, para. 1). Part of what makes this approach—athletes as agents of soft power—effective is the tribalistic bond that exists between spectators and athletes, a bond that has been studied and documented. "A huge part of who they are, where they derive a lot of their positive and negative affect, is from what their team is doing," states Edward Hirt, an associate professor of psychological and brain sciences at Indiana University Bloomington (Wang, 2006, par. 7). To fans, according to Schafer in the book, *Sociology of Sport,* their team is an "extension of their personal sense of self" (as cited in Hirt, Zillmann, Erickson, & Kennedy, pg. 725), becoming a component of the fan's self-esteem.

Athletes are symbols of their teams, a focus for fans' self-identification and self-esteem. These cultural stars are wooed by advertisers, who use their testimonials and endorsements to attract customers (soft power!) (Lamb, Hair, & McDaniel, 2011). Athletes have begun to use that power to attract support for their own policy goals, such as Dennis Rodman's trips to North Korea in pursuit of detente with that country. Rodman attempted to use his popularity and credibility as an athlete to empower a popular movement encouraging the United States to re-engage with North Korea in traditional diplomatic venues (Korostelina, 2014).

US AND IRAN IN SPORTS— PARTICIPANT PERSPECTIVES

Dennis Rodman is but the latest athlete to make waves in international diplomacy. Since 1995, Iran and the United States have met in a sporting environment over ten times, either in the States or in Iran, principally in soccer, volleyball, and wrestling. In 1998, during the time of Mohammad Khatami's presidency (1997-2005), the teams met twice: once in Iran for the Takhti Cup, an event that signified the first visit by an American sports team since the 1979 Islamic revolution. The second time was in Lyon, France, when Iran and US were paired in Group F of the FIFA World Cup, an event referenced at the start of this chapter. From 1997 through 2013, few sport exchanges between America and Iran took place, a period spanning two Iranian presidencies (Mahmoud Ahmadinejad succeeded Khatami in 2005). Many American analysts and government officials hailed Khatami as a "moderate" who made policy shifts to begin a new era of engagement with Iran. "Moderate" is, of course, a relative term and subject to misinterpretation given the differences between the U.S. and Iranian political spectra. It is, however, an objective fact that sporting exchanges failed to increase under Khatami and Ahmadinejad. It wasn't until 2013 that they began to increase in frequency, with at least eight exchanges taking place in either Iran or the US during that span. Notably, the U.S. media has dedicated significantly more attention to these events than Iranian media has.

Shared affinity for the sport has been a unifying force between wrestling officials in both countries. Rich Bender, Executive Director of USA Wrestling, states that, "Sports are a force for good. They bring people together. And interaction increases understanding and lowers barriers. Love of sports is a commonality even among nations that see things differently in terms of politics and religion" (Islamic Republic News Agency, 2013, par. 48). Mr. Bender is positive about the treatment of American athletes visiting Iran for these events, claiming that "[t]hey have been really supportive of our athletes and have cheered them on. Most U.S.-Iran interaction revolves around competitions and exchanges, with the exception of our current joint effort to keep wrestling in the 2020 Olympics" (Islamic Republic News Agency, 2013, par. 43).

In 2013, a joint effort between the Iranian, Russian, and American wrestling teams was made to promote and preserve wrestling as an Olympic sport. This trip, which began in New York and ended in Los Angeles, marked Iran's first visit to the country since 2003. Hojatollah Khatib, head of the Iranian Wrestling Federation stated that such joint efforts are important in that they demonstrate resistance against any decision to ban wrestling from the Olympics and provides for opportunities to "show our unity (Associated Press, 2013, par. 12). Khatib's statement is especially interesting given his role as a government official" (Islamic Republic of Iran Wrestling Federation, 2015). Iran's use of appointed officials in what are traditionally goodwill sporting events arguably mixes traditional and public diplomacy. The corresponding U.S. representatives are not formal members of government (*traditional* diplomats).

In response to the International Olympic Committee's decision to drop wrestling from its roster of sports, Iranian gold medalist Ali Reza Dabir linked sport to a cultural and historical aspect of society: "[D]o we destroy our historical sites which are symbols of humanity? No. Then, why should we destroy wrestling?" (Associated Press, 2013, par. 18). After the New York portion of this competition, Iranian media reported that U.S. officials would not guarantee the Iranian team's safety in Los Angeles, an assertion that a USA Wrestling spokesperson called a "total fabrication" (Wharton, 2013). State Department officials attempted to encourage team officials to continue forward to Los Angeles, which the athletes had seemed especially eager to visit since the city—nicknamed "Tehrangeles"—enjoys the largest Iranian diaspora population in the US.

Americans, both officials and athletes, were disheartened by this abrupt departure. Jordan Burroughs, a 2012 Olympic gold medalist, spoke well of the Iranian athletes, mentioning that "They don't ever wrestle dirty. Regardless if they win or lose, they shake hands with the opposing coaches and with their opponents" (Wharton, 2013, par. 15).

This same year, the International Foundation for Civil Society, with assistance from the United States Department of State and Iranian and American volleyball federations, organized a competition in Los Angeles between Iran and the US. "We see [this visit] as an incredible opportunity to promote good will and understanding between the Iranian and American people," Greg Sullivan, a senior advisor to the State Department on Iran, told

Al-Monitor (Slavin, 2014b, par. 9). Sullivan continued, that it is "part of an ongoing effort to promote exchanges in sports, arts, education and culture between the civil societies of both countries" (Slavin, 2014b, par. 9). Bahman Bakhtiari, founder of the International Foundation for Civil Society, says that the warm welcome the city and the diaspora gave the Iranian team "says a lot about the changing atmosphere" toward Iran (Slavin, 2014b, par. 5).

Several other such events have taken place, notably a volleyball competition in Tehran in 2015 that marked the first time in history the two countries' teams competed in that sport. During these exchanges, Iranian athletes are rarely quoted, while the thoughts of their American counterparts have been frequently included in media coverage. George Dill of the U.S. Polo Association says of his visit to Iran that he has never had "so much fun. The people are hospitable, friendly, the Polo is good. I encourage everyone to come here and see the country" (NBC, 2014).

Robby Smith, the number one U.S. heavyweight Greco-Roman wrestler, told Al-Monitor that the reception he got from Iranian fans during the 2014 World Cup for Greco-Roman wrestling was "the most incredible I've ever experienced" (Slavin 2014a, par. 7). The optimism surrounding the reception of both Iranian and American athletes traveling to each other's countries has extended outside of sports. Mitch Hull, the national team's Director for USA Wrestling states that "[w]e have great confidence that we can work with the Iranian Wrestling Federation, Iranian wrestlers and the Iranian people to show the world that, no matter what's happening politically, we have the same goal and the same belief and passion about the sport of wrestling" (Associated Press, 2013, par. 8).

Indeed, from the perspectives of sport officials and athletes, their experiences provide them with reason to believe that. James Ravannack, the president of USA Wrestling has said that "sports can heal a lot of politics if politicians would let us" (Slavin, 2014a, par. 24). American and Iranian athletes, administrators, and spectators, who have been a part of these exchanges over the course of different presidencies, suggest that continued engagement between parties can ultimately escalate to instantiation of policy through public diplomacy.

What these and related testimonials demonstrate is that the engagements—driven by athlete involvement—serve as a form of meaning-making. These phenomena help counter stereotypes, assumptions, and imposed or adopted worldviews. Through mass attention and the social media that is so prevalent in today's era, they penetrate the public mindset regardless of government opinion.

THEORY LINKED TO PRACTICE

Taking testimonials into consideration through observation and praxis is one thing; understanding the underlying theoretical foundation—the hows and whys of occurrences—is quite another. Theories are informed by breaking down practice, while similarly, practice helps to inform theory. It is a cyclical, mutually supportive relationship that enhances our intellectual understanding and applications. In sport diplomacy exchanges, several theories have risen to prominence.

As athletes meet, they each bring to the event their internalized worldviews. These worldviews have cultural and structural ties, and may not be consciously known by the individuals themselves. The ties form to create a narrative framework through which athletes' stories help them make sense of the world. Often, they delegitimize members of different communities, particularly when there is conflict involved. Tajfel and Turner (1979) created *social identity theory,* which states that individuals categorize themselves as belonging to a group and such labeling leads to *ingroup favoritism,* a function of comparing an *ingroup* member to one from another group, an *outgroup.* Positively distinguishing an ingroup member from an outgroup member creates a positive sense of self and increases self-esteem, all of which is defined through an us-versus-them dichotomy. We see this dichotomy in rhetoric and traditional diplomatic engagements between Iran and the US, which have focused primarily on transactional deals, positions, and interests. An us-versus-them divide can certainly be present in sport events as well, a natural consequence of the zero-sum nature of competitions. Exchanges can, and fortunately do, occur during these events and can focus on cooperative forces, encouraging participants to work together toward a similar goal that can transcend the zero-sum dynamic.

To begin to overcome such a dynamic, we can look to the criterion proposed by Gordon Allport's *intergroup contact theory* (Allport, 1954). The premise of this theory states that interpersonal contact between groups, particularly between majority and minority group members, is one of the most effective ways to reduce prejudice. The opportunity to engage provides a platform through which participants can communicate and try to understand the other's way of life; contact increases understanding and, if sustained, can lead to reduced prejudice and stereotyping. An environment that is structured around cooperation, controlled for the least amount of differences, and includes a shared common goal, personal interaction, and support of some entity from both sides will raise the chances of yielding friendly experiences that bridge divides (Allport, 1954).

We see traces of these theories playing out in the sport exchanges between the Americans and Iranians. Stereotyping, prejudices, and one group pitted against the other (us versus them) were all present yet the testimonial samples provide evidence that athletes and officials alike were able to see beyond the commonplace narratives they first harbored going into the exchanges. Teams were well-received by the host country, positive character and skills-related comments were made, and visiting athletes had such positive experiences that they encouraged others to visit as well. These experiences help to disseminate new messages, begin building new narratives, and serve as a means to legitimize—rather than dehumanize—the "other."

BEYOND BREAKING THE ICE: A NEW AGE

Traditional diplomacy, which involves hard power, does not reflect public opinion. It creates deals, negotiations, and barriers that may not be visible to the public. Diplomats have been the traditional carriers of this track of diplomacy and this practice is today becoming increasingly defunct and ineffective (at least in this context). For the past 60 years, the US and Iran have enjoyed mostly a stalemate; neither government achieving their diplomatic goals without conceding too much.

Public diplomacy, on the other hand, involves the communication of peoples of one community with those of another. It is about engagement, attraction, and cooperation. More so, it is increasingly gaining traction in today's information-driven, global era. Its benefits lie in connecting nongovernment actors who would otherwise be excluded from negotiations and policy conversations and agenda; and its downfall comes from exactly the fact that it connects a large amount and range of opinion that are both relevant and irrelevant to diplomacy.

With this expansion of influence, athletes cannot be ignored. They are indeed a publicly visible focus within events that are cultural in nature and more often than not have very little to do with traditional diplomacy. In the case of the US-Iran conflict, athletes have continued to come together and demonstrate the ability and desire to compete with one another and test their skills while expressing respect and sportsmanship. They have also done so irrespective of each government's negative, and at times demonizing, opinions of the other—something that traditional diplomacy has lost. Blocking such engagement by traditional diplomacy, hasty action becomes foolish; take, for example, the Iranian team's swift and mysterious departure after the New York promotional wrestling match.

As public diplomacy actors, athletes can communicate messages that traditional diplomacy cannot, positioning them to ensure that messages are coming across. They do so through tapping into the publics (the *populi* of Rome mentioned earlier) of different communities—the fans, the players, and their larger respective communities with whom they will share their experiences. The effect is enhanced by social media platforms, creating an enduring impact beyond the actual events because the connections between various sectors of society have been made. Athletes are agents that first connect communities and start communications between them. One way or another, these soft-power methods are going to continue. It is up to organizations that facilitate sport exchanges to make sure they maximize building bridges of cooperation and making meaning, both directly stemming from people-to-people interactions.

Organizations are the lynchpin that connects athletes with communities. They must therefore be supportive to keep this channel open and maximize opportunities that help athletes develop new narratives through constructive dialogue and teamwork activities. Athletes who want to participate in sport exchanges must have access to resources to enable them to continue these initiatives, such as private conferences, pre- and post-game meetings that encourage networking, and goodwill games with teams composed of different nationalities. In the case of Dennis Rodman, he only worked with the tools he knew; he interacted with Kim Jung Un as though he was another athlete instead of a head of a state. Consequently, the US considered him an opportunist, not an agent capable of helping to melt the ice and build lasting public diplomacy goals, or even of designing their interactions to align them with U.S. foreign policy goals for that matter.

Organizations that facilitate sport exchanges should not only recognize that the new age involves maximizing soft-power relations—of which athletes are a powerful agent—but should also position themselves to empower athletes. Empowering in this sense means helping athletes to maximize their people-to-people interactions, to spread messages that express a relatable narrative or position that makes meaning across several layers of society. Traditional diplomacy and hard power that coerce and the agents of that diplomacy and power—usually government actors such as diplomats—simply do not have the means or power to do so in the new age to the same extent that informed, socially active athletes can invoke.

The lay of the land has indeed changed. Athletes now have, through social media and networks, both the ability and platforms on which to build networks, and not just a collection of photo ops. Utilizing these tools creates avenues for the development of relationships that have the ability to build bridges among communities, resonating with people's sense of belonging, relatability, and broadening their voices. These relationships spark processes driven by stories of people-power with increased amounts of visibility. This is the new method of winning hearts and minds, one which today's athletes can propel beyond acts that simply break the ice. When athletes and channels reach a social critical mass, they can no longer be ignored by government, media, or society at large.

After sitting in the Stade Gerland in France in 1998 to watch the Iranian and American soccer teams, I was deeply affected by how one act, one event, was leveraged to communicate a political message. For me, that event did more than break the ice; it began an ongoing process of exploration as an athlete, student, and member of society. Had this act taken place in the current information age, with the support of the athletes themselves, the result would have been a completely different ball game.

DISCUSSION QUESTIONS

1. Name examples of public diplomacy efforts.
2. What is the difference between traditional and public diplomacy?
3. What prompted the transition from traditional to public diplomacy?
4. Identify some strengths and weaknesses of soft power. Where have you seen them at play?
5. Identify athletes who have affected American society in some shape or form?
6. How can athletes act as soft power agents?
7. What are some group dynamics to be cognizant of in sport exchanges?
8. What is a real-world example of a scenario in which soft power succeeded after hard power failed?
9. Explain the role of sport in Iranian and American society.
10. In what ways can organizations that create sport exchanges maximize positive athlete-to-athlete interaction?

REFERENCES

Abrahamian, E. (1982). *Iran between two revolutions*. Princeton, NJ: Princeton University Press.

Allport, G. W. (1954). *The nature of prejudice*. Cambridge, MA: Perseus Books.

Arquila, J., & Ronfeldt, D. (1999). *The emergence of neopolitik: Toward an American information strategy*. Santa Monica, CA: RAND.

Aspen Institute. (2015). *Sport for all: Play for life. A playbook to get every kid in the game*. Washington, DC.: Aspen Institute.

Associated Press. (2013). Iran-US wrestling match in Los Angeles cancelled. Retrieved from http://www.nydailynews.com/news/world/iran-find-common-ground-olympic-wrestling-article-1.1267811

Aviel, J. F. (2005). The evolution of multilateral diplomacy. In J. P. Muldoon Jr., J. F. Aviel, R. Reitano, & E. Sullivan (Eds.), *Multilateral diplomacy and the United Nations today* (pp. 15-22). Cambridge, MA: Westview Press.

Avruch, K. (2013). *Context and pretext in conflict resolution: Culture, identity, power, and practice*. Boulder, CO: Paradigm Publishers.

Billings, A. C., Butterworth, M. L., & Turman, P. D. (2015). *Communication and sport: Surveying the field*. New York, NY: Sage Publications, Inc.

Block, D. (2005). *Baseball before we knew it: A search for the roots of the game*. Lincoln, NE: University of Nebraska Press.

Brower, C. N., & Brueschke, J. D. (1998). *The Iran-United States claims tribunal*. The Hague, Netherlands: Martinus Nijhoff Publishers.

Brumberg, D. (2001). *Reinventing Khomeini: The struggle for reform in Iran*. Chicago, IL: University of Chicago Press.

Bull, H. (1977). *The anarchical society: A study of order in world politics*. New York, NY: Columbia University Press.

Byrne, M. (2015). *Iran and the United States in the cold war*. Retrieved from https://www.gilderlehrman.org/history-by-era/age-reagan/essays/iran-and-united-states-cold-war

Byrne, M., & Gasiorowski, M. J. (2004). *Mohammad Mosaddeq and the 1953 coup in Iran*. Syracuse, NY: Syracuse University Press.

Chehabi, H. E. (2002). The juggernaut of globalization: Sport and modernization in Iran. The *International Journal of the History of Sport, 19*, 275-294.

Chehabi, H. E. (1995). Sport and politics in Iran: The legend of Gholamreza Takhti. *International Journal of the History of Sport, 12*(3), 48-60.

Choksy, C. E, & Choksy, J. K. (2015). *The Saudi connection: Wahhabism and global jihad*. Retrieved from http://www.worldaffairsjournal.org/article/saudi-connection-wahhabism-and-global-jihad

Clawson, P. (2010). U.S. sanctions. In R. Wright (Ed.), *The Iran primer: Power, politics, and U.S. policy* (115-118). Washington, D.C.: United States Institute of Peace.

Cordesman, A. H., & Al-Rodhan, K. R. (2006). *Iran's weapons of mass destruction: The real and potential threat*. Washington, D.C.: CSIS Press.

Dabashi, H. (2008). *Islamic liberation theology: Resisting the empire*. New York, NY: Routledge.

Daugherty, W. (2003). *Jimmy Carter and the 1979 decision to admit the Shah in the United States*. Retrieved from http://www.unc.edu/depts/diplomat/archives_roll/2003_01-03/dauherty_shah/dauherty_shah.html

Elias, R. (2011). *Baseball and American foreign policy*. Retrieved from https://transatlantica.revues.org/5478#tocto1n8

Evans G., & Grant B. (1995). *Australia's foreign relations in the world of the 1990s*. Melbourne, AUS: Melbourne University Press.

Farber, D. (2005). *Taken hostage: The Iran hostage crisis and America's first encounter with radical Islam*. Princeton, NJ: Princeton University Press.

Gregory, B. (2014). *The paradox of US public diplomacy: Its rise and "demise."* Retrieved from https://ipdgc.gwu.edu/sites/ipdgc.gwu.edu/files/downloads/IPDGC-SpecialReport1-BGregory.pdf

Guttman, A. (2007). *Sports: The first five millennia*. Boston, MA: University of Massachusetts Press.

Hill, J.B. (2007). *Robinson affected American society: Robinson's efforts led to changes in America*. Retrieved from http://m.mlb.com/news/article/1898206/

Hirt, E. R., Zillmann, D., Erickson, G. A., & Kennedy, C. (1992). Costs and benefits of allegiance: Changes in fans' self-ascribed competencies after team victory versus defeat. *Journal of Personality and Social Psychology, 63,* 724-738.

Ignatius, D. (2015). The paradox of Pope Francis's power. Retrieved from https://www.washingtonpost.com/opinions/the-paradox-of-the-popes-power/2015/09/24/9533401a-62ca-11e5-b38e-06883aacba64_story.html

Islamic Republic of Iran Wrestling Federation (2015). Khatib selects as temporary headman of Iran Wrestling Federation. Retrieved from http://webcache.googleusercontent.com/search?q=cache:cCMkUFZsxzoJ:en.iawf.ir/Content/Content.aspx%3FMode%3D1%26PageCode%3D28090+&cd=6&hl=en&ct=clnk&gl=us

Kiani, M. G., & Faraji, H. (2011). Zoorkhaneh: Historic training in Iranian culture. *World Applied Sciences Journal, 14,* 1415-1423.

Korostelina, K. (2014). *Political insults: How offenses escalate conflict*. Oxford, UK: Oxford University Press.

Kressin, W.K. (1991). Prime minister Mossadegh and Ayatollah Kashani from unity to enmity: As viewed from the American embassy in Tehran, June 1950-August 1953. Retrieved from http://www.dtic.mil/dtic/tr/fulltext/u2/a239339.pdf

Lamb, C., Hair, J., & McDaniel, C. (2011). *Essentials of marketing*. Boston, MA: Cengage Learning.

Limbert, J. (2009). *Negotiating with Iran: Wrestling the ghosts of history*. Washington, D.C.: United States Institute of Peace.

Morello, C. (2015). Another Iranian American arrested and imprisoned in Tehran. Retrieved from https://www.washingtonpost.com/world/national-security/another-iranian-american-arrested-and-imprisoned-in-tehran/2015/10/29/8d540056-7999-11e5-b9c1-f03c48c96ac2_story.html

Morris, P. (2006). *A game of inches: The stories behind the innovations that shaped baseball*. Chicago, IL: Ivan R. Dee.

Murray, S. (2012). Sports diplomacy: A hybrid of two halves. Retrieved from http://www.cultural-diplomacy.org/academy/content/pdf/participant-papers/2011-symposium/Sports-Diplomacy-a-hybrid-of-two-halves--Dr-Stuart-Murray.pdf

National Broadcasting Company (NBC). (2014). Polo diplomacy: U.S. players travel to Iran to horse around. Retrieved from http://www.nbcnews.com/watch/nbc-news/polo-diplomacy-u-s-players-travel-to-iran-to-horse-around-276908611836

Nye, J. (2003). *The paradox of American power: Why the world's only superpower can't go it alone*. Oxford, UK: Oxford University Press.

Nye, J. (2006). Smart power: In search of the balance between hard and soft power. *Democracy: A Journal of Ideas. 2,* 85-90.

Nye, J. (2008). Public diplomacy and soft power. *The American Academy of Political and Social Science 616*(1), 94-109.

Islamic Republic News Agency. (2013). Iran-US wrestling match in Los Angeles cancelled. Retrieved from http://www.payvand.com/news/13/may/1134.html

President's Council on Fitness, Sports & Nutrition. (2015). Our mission. Retrieved from http://www.fitness.gov/about-pcfsn/our-mission-and-vision/

Rahnema, A. (2015). *Behind the 1953 coup in Iran: Thugs, turncoats, soldiers, and spooks*. Cambridge, UK: Cambridge University Press.

Reiss, S. (1999). *Touching base: Professional baseball and American culture in the progressive era*. Champaign, IL: University of Illinois Press.

Samore, Gary. (2015). The Iran nuclear deal: A definitive guide. Retrieved from http://belfercenter.ksg.harvard.edu/files/IranDealDefinitiveGuide.pdf?webSyncID=481969e1-d6e1-01d6-9107-7657215a1003&sessionGUID=9e1b2808-6ac0-b0b9-565e-d7b6411031c5

Sandre, A. (2013). Twitter for diplomats. Retrieved from http://issuu.com/diplo/docs/twitter_for_diplomats

Schafer, W E. (1969). Some sources and consequences of interscholastic athletics. In G. S. Kenyon (Ed.), *Sociology of sport*. Chicago: Athletic Institute.

Segell, G. (2005). *Axis of evil and rogue states: The Bush administration, 2000-2004*. London, UK: Glen Segell.

Simon, H. A. (1998). Information 101: It's not what you know, it's how you know it. *Journal for Quality and Participation 21* (4), 30-33.

Simon, H. A. (1971). Designing organizations for an information rich world. In D. Greenberger, *Computers, Communication, and the Public Interest* (pp. 38-72). Baltimore, MD: Johns Hopkins Press.

Slavin, B. (2014a). American athletes get star treatment in Iran. Retrieved from http://www.al-monitor.com/pulse/originals/2014/07/us-athletes-diplomacy-iran.html#

Slavin, B. (2014b). Iran, US try volleyball diplomacy. Retrieved from http://www.al-monitor.com/pulse/ru/originals/2014/08/iran-volleyball-team-united-states-sports-diplomacy.html#

Tajfel, H., & Turner, J. C. (1979). An integrative theory of intergroup conflict. In W. G. Austin & S. Worchel (Eds.), *The social psychology of intergroup relations*. Monterey, CA: Brooks-Cole.

Tyson, A.S. (2005). Iran protests U.S. aerial drones. Retrieved from http://www.washingtonpost.com/wp-dyn/content/article/2005/11/07/AR2005110701450.html

United States Government. (2006). *Congressional record: Proceedings and debates of the 109th Congress second session*. Washington, D.C.: United States Government Printing Office.

United States Department of State. (2016). Under secretary for public diplomacy and public affairs. Retrieved from http://www.state.gov/r/

United States Department of State, Bureau of Educational and Cultural Affairs. (2016). Programs and initiatives. Retrieved from http://eca.state.gov/programs-initiatives/sports-diplomacy

von Clausewitz, C. (1918). On war (Col. J. J. Graham, Trans.). London, UK: Kegan Paul, Trench, Trubner & Company.

Wang, S. (2006). Sports complex: The science behind fanatic behavior. *Observer 19* (5). Retrieved from http://www.psychologicalscience.org/index.php/publications/observer/2006/may-06/sports-complex-the-science-behind-fanatic-behavior.html

Wharton, D. (2013). Iran's wrestling team abruptly decides to skip L.A. competition. Retrieved from http://articles.latimes.com/2013/may/17/sports/la-sp-us-iran-wrestling-20130518

Woollacott, M. (2002). 'Soft power' can win the battle for hearts and minds. The Guardian. Retrieved from http://www.theguardian.com/politics/2002/aug/02/usa.world

Zakeri, M. (1995). *Sasanid soldiers in early Muslim society: The origins of 'Ayyārān and Futuwwa*. Weisbaden, GER: Harrassowitz Verlag.

10

FROM CANADA WITH LOVE: HUMAN RIGHTS, SOFT POWER, AND THE PRIDE HOUSE MOVEMENT

KYLE RICH · LAURA MISENER

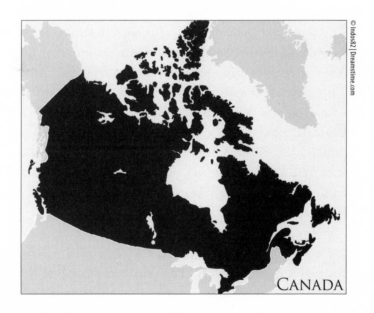

CANADA

"There's no place for the state in the bedrooms of the nation."

The quote above was spoken by Canadian Justice Minister (and eventually Prime Minister) Pierre Trudeau after introducing the Omnibus bill, which would change the legal landscape of sexuality in Canada, in the House of Commons on December 21, 1967 (CBC, 1967). The bill proposed serious amendments to the criminal code, which would decriminalize homosexuality in Canada by way of relaxing laws around sexual activity between consenting adults. The introduction of this bill, often embodied in these words, represents an important point in history for the rights of lesbian, gay, bisexual, trans, queer (LGBTQ[1]) and two-spirited[2]-identified persons and communities in Canada. Indeed, this bill became a platform from which many legislative changes began and continue to emerge.

Despite nearly 50 years of political attention, the struggle for equal rights of LGBTQ-identified persons continues in Canada. Recently, sport has become prominent in these discussions and a vehicle through which political attention and social change is being sought. The emergence of organizations and initiatives such as the You Can Play Project (You Can Play, n.d.) and the Canadian Olympic Committee's #OneTeam initiative (Canadian Olympic Committee, n.d.) have recently brought attention to issues surrounding homophobia in sport and the need for strategic efforts to change the culture and norms of sporting activities from the grassroots to elite levels. With the attention and support of elite level athletes, discussions about LGBTQ-identified persons and athletes have become prominent in the media and to some extent public discourse. Recently, these trends are exemplified by several high-profile international athletes coming out at various stages of their career (e.g., former Olympians Ian Thorpe, and Caitlyn Jenner, NFL draft pick Michael Sam, NBA player Jason Collins, and current Olympians Gus Kenworthy, Eric Radford, Rose Cossar, and Connor Taras). These announcements drew extensive media attention and further integrated sport into discussions around experiences of LGBTQ-identified (and closeted) people in sport and society more broadly (e.g., see Cox, 2015). Thus, while the struggles for LGBTQ equality are not new in Canada, the existence of a role for sport to play in this diplomatic endeavour is relatively recent. In this chapter, we address the notion of sport diplomacy in the context of advancing the LGBTQ acceptance and integration in sport and society in general. The conjuncture will be explored through the example of the Pride House Movement, developments, and event-related operations in the Canadian context.

During the Vancouver 2010 Winter Olympic Games, the first Pride House pavilions were organized as welcoming spaces for LGBTQ folks and allies. Pavilions in Vancouver and Whistler, as well as the QMUNITY Centre on Davie Street (Vancouver's LGBTQ community hub) hosted over 20,000 visitors and garnered significant media attention, acknowledged in the legacy report as the third most reported story of the Games (Birch-Jones, 2010). Just five years later, the movement has grown exponentially, using a number of major games (e.g., London 2012 Olympic Games, FIFA 2014 World Cup and Rio 2016 Olympic Games in Brazil, Glasgow 2014 Commonwealth Games, and Toronto 2015 Pan/Parapan American Games) as platforms to advance discussions around sexual orientation and gender identity in and through sport. The recent edition, PridehouseTO, is described as "a comprehensive, province-wide engagement and activation strategy for [LGBTQ] communities," initiated to "leverage the TORONTO 2015 Pan/Parapan Am Games to build a stronger, healthier society" (PridehouseTO, 2015a, para 1). Despite being a relatively young organization, the Pridehouse Movement has experienced significant growth and gained much attention in Canada and internationally. In this chapter, we examine the strategies developed and employed in Vancouver/Whistler (2010) and in Toronto (2015). Using the concept of soft power, we assess the potential of these sport-based strategies as critical diplomatic tools in eliciting social change for LGBTQ communities. We begin with an overview of the Canadian context, specifically with regards to public policy and the rights of LGBTQ-identified persons as this sets the stage for diplomatic opportunities associated with human rights. Next, we draw upon the theoretical constructs of leveraging sport events and soft power to situate how the LGBTQ community and Pride House sought to capitalize on the opportunity provided by major games to address broader issues of social inclusion, both in Canada and abroad. Third, we review the strategies developed and employed by PRIDEhouse (Vancouver) and PridehouseTO (Toronto) in order to assess their diplomatic potential and how they may influence discussions and the realizing of sexual rights in diverse contexts. Finally, we conclude with a commentary on the potential of using sport for diplomatic purposes in the Canadian context and abroad.

CANADIAN VALUES AND PUBLIC POLICY

Defining and articulating Canadian culture and values are not easy tasks. Across the enormous land mass there exists vastly diverse geographic, social, and political contexts. Indeed, in his sweeping historical examination of Canadian culture, Vance (2009) describes Canada as a place of unparalleled diversity. Populations include indigenous, settler, and more recently immigrated inhabitants dispersed in various patterns across urban, rural, and remote communities. The result is a complex diaspora of communities with vastly different lived experiences and perspectives. However, Jackson (1998) notes that "where struggles occur with respect to the politics of media representation, there is a tendency to define collective identities, including national ones, as distinct, fully constituted entities" (p. 229). Indeed, in an era of globalization and technology, there exist mediated and often paradoxical (at least from a Canadian perspective) stereotypes of Canada, in which sport features prominently: a rugged northern territory populated with diverse, socially progressive, rural-dwelling hockey players. For example, one need only consider images of Canadian NHL superstar, Sidney Crosby, as a young boy playing "Timbits hockey" (an introductory hockey program funded by the Canadian coffee shop franchise named after former NHL player Tim Horton) in Coal Harbour, Nova Scotia. These images depict a "typical" Canadian experience, and are notoriously given airtime during the annual IIHF World Junior Hockey Championship (a tournament with which the Canadian media has an ostensible obsession). Another example can be viewed in the recently released Canadian Olympic Committee campaign called "Ice in Our Veins" which highlights Canadian Olympic athletes training for the 2016 Rio Olympic Games. These athletes are depicted training for their summer sports in rugged arctic landscapes. These representations conjure up images of what is presented as *the* Canadian youth experience. However, as noted by Wilson (2006), while hockey remains an important symbol of national pride and community in Canada, globalization and diverse cultural influences are creating much more diverse Canadian experiences and youth culture(s). While these mythical images are clearly not universally applicable, they demonstrate that Canadian culture is one of diversity: diverse contexts, diverse populations, and diverse landscapes, which in turn allow for a plethora of diverse cultures and communities to emerge.

PUBLIC POLICY AND DIVERSITY IN CANADA

Public policy in Canada has (for the most part) aligned with the image and culture of diversity. Examples of this can be found in regards to multiculturalism, healthcare, indigenous rights, and sexual orientation and gender identity (which will be addressed more thoroughly in the following section). In regards to multiculturalism, Banting and Kymlicka (2010) identify two policy changes that officially shifted Canada away from a discriminatory and assimilationist approach to ethnicity. First was the adoption of the points system—a race neutral admission criterion—to immigration in 1967. Second was the adoption of the multiculturalism policy in 1971, making Canada the first country in the world to adopt an official policy of the sort (Government of Canada, 2012). Since that time, the Canadian government has been committed to recognizing and accommodating diversity, removing barriers to being full participants in society, promoting the building of relationships and exchange between groups, and the promotion of the official languages (i.e., French and English; Banting & Kymlicka, 2010). While space does not permit us to elaborate fully, it should be noted that Canada's approach to multiculturalism is important, with wide-reaching implications, because it involves many political and historical issues, including but not limited to those related to Aboriginal peoples, Québecois nationalism, and recent changes in immigration patterns.

An example that resonates and applies to all Canadians (particularly in comparison to our neighbours from the south) is the publicly funded healthcare system that provides universal coverage and access to care. This model is one of which Canadians are proud and likely to defend in comparison to two-tiered or private systems (Mendelsohn, 2002). Universal healthcare is often presented as symbolic of the value Canadians place on diversity and acceptance. Indeed, Health Canada notes that "the principles governing our healthcare system are symbols of the underlying Canadian values of equity and solidarity" (Health Canada, 2010, para. 1). Healthcare in the Canadian context is thus presented as an example of effective alignment of public policy with underlying values.

Conversely, an area of policy that may be considered misaligned with Canadian values of equity and solidarity would be policies that engage Aboriginal peoples in Canada.[4] Indigenous groups of Canada include First Nations, Inuit, and Métis peoples. These groups have been historically mistreated and disrespected through processes of colonization and attempts at assimilation, clearly illustrated through examples such as the residential schooling system, which was not fully shut down until the 1990s (Indigenous and Northern Affairs Canada, 2014). Historically, there are numerous policies regarding the treatment of Aboriginal peoples, notably *The Indian Act* (Government of Canada, 1985), which was

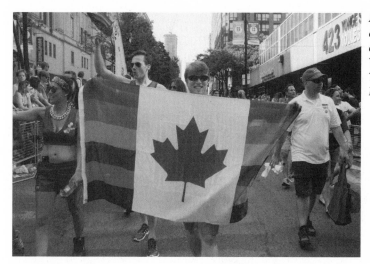

A PridehouseTO ambassador carrying a flag during the 2014 WorldPride Parade in Toronto. Photo courtesy of Patti Anne Valenti.

first introduced in 1876. More recently, concern with the political treatment of Aboriginal peoples in Canada has become part of public discourse, aided by activist movements (e.g., Idle No More) as well as political endeavours such as the Truth and Reconciliation Commission (Truth and Reconciliation Commission of Canada, 2015). These changes may be represented by Prime Minister Harper's historic (albeit paradoxical, based on other changes made under the Harper Government) apology to individuals and families implicated in the residential school system (Indigenous and Northern Affairs Canada, 2014). These changes suggest shifting political and public concern with issues surrounding Aboriginal peoples in Canada. While late to the game, perhaps these shifting political concerns represent the beginning of what may be an attempt by the federal government to better align policies (that have historically been assimilationist and discriminatory) with so-called Canadian values.

SEXUAL RIGHTS AND PUBLIC POLICY

In Canada and internationally, sexual orientation and gender identity have an interesting relationship with public policy at many levels. Despite documents outlining the tensions and gaps (internationally) in human rights and rights of LGBTQ-identified persons (see Declaration of Montreal, 2006, and the Yogyakarta Principles, 2007), when taken up by multinational organizations, the topic has been embraced in some policy agendas and not others. Swiebel (2009) explores the discussions of sexual rights at the United Nations (UN) and European Union (EU). She uses agenda-setting and social movement theory to describe the implications of mobilizing structures (i.e., resources and points of access into an organization), issue framing (i.e., sexual rights versus human rights), and political opportunity structures (notably friendly elites who offer support) on how issues of sexual rights have been taken up at these fora. Consequently, she attributes existing structures and support as well as a human rights framing of the issues to the success of the conversations that took place at the EU, which can be starkly contrasted with the UN, where "although the circle of 'friendly elites' is growing, they are not numerous or strong enough to outweigh opposing forces from (mainly) Islamist and conservative Catholic states and NGOs" (Swiebel, 2009, p. 29). Based on these observations, it is clear the governing bodies around the world have vastly different values and approaches to the rights of LGBTQ-identified persons, making it a site where exchange and learning have the potential to elicit meaningful dialogue and drive change, if addressed strategically.

In Canada, discussions and public policy regarding sexual orientation and gender identity have made dramatic progress since the introduction of the Omnibus bill in 1967. Importantly, these changes should not be seen in a vacuum but rather as complementary to other public policy developments such as multiculturalism policy (discussed above) as well as the Canadian Charter of Rights and Freedoms, which was introduced in 1982 recognizing that all individuals are "equal before and under the law and ha[ve] the right to the equal protection and equal benefit of the law without discrimination" (Government of Canada, 1982, section 15, para. 1). Indeed, Smith (1999) discussed the implications of the Charter in shaping the political action in LGBTQ communities, transforming it from "liberation" in the 1970s to a human rights-focused movement in the 1980s and 1990s. In restricting our overview to the development of public policy in Canada, we might consider the following major milestones: (a) the federal government passing (after several prior attempts) Bill C-33, which included sexual orientation in the Canadian Human Rights Act in 1996; (b) the Supreme Court of Canada ruling that same-sex couples should have the same rights as opposite-sex common-law couples in 1999 and the subsequent passage of Bill C-23 allowing them that right in 2000; (c) the Ontario Court of Appeals upholding a ruling to allow same sex marriage (with the first ceremony taking place the same day as the ruling) and several other provinces following suit in 2003; and finally, (d) the Senate's approval of Bill C-38 giving same sex couples the right to marry in 2005, making Canada the fourth country in the world to do so (CBC, 2012[5]). More recently, considerations around gender identity are also finding their way into public policy. In 2015, a surprise move by Citizenship and Immigration Canada removed the requirement for proof of sex reassignment surgery when individuals are asking to change the sex designation on their citizenship certificates (Citizenship and Immigration Canada, 2015). This change "puts the federal requirements more in line with provinces, where change is swiftly spreading across the country" and is an important step towards the right to self-identify (Strapagiel, 2015, para. 5). Provincially, many jurisdictions are in the process of amending laws that will ease the process for individuals asking to change their sex on birth certificates (Canadian Civil Liberties Association, 2015) as well as providing better access and shorter wait times for sex reassignment surgery (Leslie, 2015). As public policy has many implications for LGBTQ-identified (and closeted) persons, the current situation is far from perfect. However, it should be noted that nationally and provincially, Canadian governments are actively engaged in discussions about sexual orientation and gender identity. While the ebbs and flows of change are undoubtedly influenced by

changes in governments, the last decade has shown consistent progress towards a more
robust recognition of sexual rights in Canada.

Against this backdrop, we will now shift our focus to discussing the role of sport in
advancing this public policy agenda in Canada and abroad. By considering the role of major
sports events as a form of sport diplomacy, we consider the Pride House movement as a
cultural export emanating from Canadian host cities. Using the notion of soft power (Nye,
2008), we discuss how the movement may potentially be a way of realizing the human
rights of LGBTQ-identified persons throughout Canada and around the world.

SPORT EVENTS AND SOFT POWER

Within the study of public diplomacy, soft power has become a prominent lens through
which to discuss international relations and policy (Rothman, 2011). Soft power can be
understood as 'attractive power' or the ways in which groups, organizations, or nations get
others to want what they want, without the use of coercion (Nye, 2008). In the context of
international relations, Nye (2008) notes that soft power also necessitates an alignment of
public policy with values of the nation, as well as the nature of the relationships with other
countries. Within the context of sport, Nygård and Gates (2013) identified four mechanisms
of soft power: image-building; building a platform for dialogue; trust building; and reconciliation, integration, and anti-racism. An emerging literature pertaining to soft power in the
context of sport involves the use of large-scale sporting events (e.g., the Olympic Games or
the FIFA World Cup) for countries to establish themselves as emerging powers in an increasingly globalized world (e.g., see Gulianotti, 2015; Grix & Houlihan, 2014).

Large-scale events offer the space for engaging in discussions of power, politics, and
broader issues of diplomacy. Scholars have suggested that liminal spaces created around
events, such as festivals and sporting events, suspend typical social hierarchies, allowing
for the creation of new social spaces that can be engaged to generate discussion and address
issues, effectively eliciting social change (Chalip, 2006; Grix, 2015). Events present an
opportunity through which host countries and organizations therein attempt to use the liminal spaces created around the event for social, cultural, and economic outcomes. Leveraging
efforts strategically attempt to accomplish a variety of outcomes, including increased revenue generation, tourism, sport participation, and the changing of attitudes and awareness
of certain issues (Misener, McGillivray, McPherson, & Legg, 2015; Taks, Green, Misener, &
Chalip, 2014). The concept of using events for social change is not new per se, as evidenced
by famous political acts such as the black power salute of Tommie Smith and John Carlos at
the 1968 Olympic Games, or the boycotts of the 1980 and 1984 Games; however embracing
the event as a strategic opportunity to influence broader social and political agendas has
given rise to new political platforms.

Nygard and Gates (2013) have argued that sport events produce numerous intended and
unintended political outcomes. It is the mechanisms associated with the event that reinforce
or produce the soft-power narratives. In effect, the importance of creating a platform for

dialogue about particularly potent political issues is at the heart of the Pride House Movement in Canada. The creation of social spaces that can be strategically leveraged to highlight inequalities, promote new social ideologies, and advance political agendas is key to not only influencing foreign policy agendas but also advancing opportunities for furthering internal political struggles. The concept of social leverage as advanced by scholars such as Chalip (2006), Schulenkorf (2010), and Misener and Schulenkorf (2016) suggest that events can be effectively utilized to advance new social ideologies. The Pride House Movement is one such strategic agenda that emerged in response to social and political inequities in a nation-state that has relatively progressive social policies for advancing the rights of the LGBTQ community.

✳ THE PRIDE HOUSE MOVEMENT

Since the 2010 edition of the Winter Olympic and Paralympic Games, Pride Houses have provided safe and welcoming spaces for LGBTQ-identified persons and allies during large, international sport events. Based on the hospitality house model (typically organized as social spaces around nationalities or cultures), Pride Houses are organized to serve demographics that are often excluded from sport spaces (Elling & Janssens, 2009) as well as from the perceived prestige of participating in international competitions. As noted on the Pride House International website:

> LGBTIQ+ people have traditionally been pushed to the margins of sport. Negative stereotypes, the threat of real and perceived consequences for living openly, and an exclusionary or hostile culture have made sport unwelcoming. . . . During large-scale international events, there is the possibility to connect with people from different cultures and backgrounds, to learn empathy and experience diversity, and to share a common appreciation for excellence. When LGBTIQ+ people are excluded, LGBTIQ+ culture is also excluded. (Pridehouse International, 2015a, para. 2)

Therefore, by using large-scale sport events as platforms, the movement seeks to foster inclusion, acceptance, and celebration of LGBTQ-identified persons and cultures in sporting contexts of host countries and internationally. While a typical Pride House includes "welcoming places to view the competitions, experience the event with others, learn about LGBTIQ+ sport and homophobia in sport, and build a relationship with mainstream sport" (Pride House International, 2015a, para. 3), the movement recognizes the importance of local social and political contexts in relation to their activities. For example, although the application to host a Pride House at the 2014 Sochi Olympic and Paralympic Games was denied (in the context of Russia's flagrantly homophobic laws leading up to the games and the International Olympic Committee's [IOC] subsequent reluctance to act on the issue), this platform allowed for the staging of a series of international remote Pride Houses and demonstrations where people could participate in solidarity with Russian LGBTQ-identified persons (Pride House International, 2015b). Furthermore, it was the events surrounding Sochi 2014 that led to the formation of Pride House International as "a coalition of LGBT sport and human rights groups, including participants in past and future Pride Houses" (Pride House International, 2015a, para. 6), that gave coherency and continuance to the movement. While the history of the movement is not long, the diverse and strategic activities undertaken appear to have generated discussions and awareness of issues surrounding sexual orientation and gender identity (in sport and more broadly) at local, state, and global levels. While Pride Houses have been hosted in several countries, we will focus our discussion on the strategies enacted in Canada, the birthplace of the Pride House Movement.

PRIDE HOUSE IN CANADA

The inaugural Pride Houses, staged in Vancouver and Whistler in 2010, were largely a result of the work and leadership of Dean Nelson. These houses were designed with several goals and outcomes in mind: creating safe spaces to unite LGBTQ communities during the games (e.g., games viewing, social events); educating, raising awareness, and evoking change around homophobia in sport and human rights more broadly (e.g., by working with Canadian sport organizations such as AthletesCAN and the Canadian Olympic Committee); and offering resources and support for LGBTQ-identified and closeted persons whose rights may not be fully recognized in other contexts (e.g., in partnership with LEGIT and Rainbow Refuge); and by celebrating queer culture through art, film nights, and various programming (Birch-Jones, 2010). Given their involvement in international relations, what is particularly interesting for our discussion are the education and outreach initiatives that attempted to raise awareness about homophobia (particularly in sport) and provide refugee and asylum support services. Indeed, it is noted in the *PRIDEhouse Legacy Report* that

> PRIDE house was intended to be significant especially to citizens from nations such as India, Iran, Jamaica, Ukraine, and 65+ other countries where it is still ILLEGAL to be a homosexual and in over 7 countries where the crime of being gay or thought to be gay is punishable by DEATH. (Birch-Jones, 2010, p. 2)

Thus, inaugural Pride Houses were not only conceived to provide safe, welcoming, and celebratory spaces for queer individuals, groups, and families, but also to demonstrate and raise awareness about Canadian values and public policy regarding sexual rights: "It is not widely known that Canada has recognized same-sex partnerships for immigration and has, for over a decade, provided refugee protection to persecuted LGBT persons" (Birch-Jones, 2010, p. 12). Although celebratory spaces and flashy pins were the most common images circulated, the underlying diplomatic endeavours were also clearly articulated, for example by Philip Steenkamp (CEO of the British Columbia Olympic and Paralympic Games Secretariat): "Really we want to celebrate our diversity and the tolerance of our culture and also showcase that to the world. . . those Canadian values of tolerance and diversity and what creates such a strength in our culture here" (cited in Kitching, 2010, para. 8). Therefore, while on the surface Pride Houses may appear to be simple celebratory spaces (as are many other hospitality houses), they also represent an important diplomatic initiative. Indeed, the goal of achieving equitable human rights for LGBTQ-identified persons internationally has been central to the purpose of the Pride House Movement since its inception.

The second Canadian installment of Pride House in Canada took place during the 2015 Pan/Parapan American Games in Toronto. This time, more lead time, organizational learning, and an extensive partnership scheme allowed the initiative to secure public funding and private sponsorship to stage strategic, multisectorial initiatives that spanned several years leading up to the games. The initiatives involved five 'projects': Pridehouse Pavillion, Education, Arts & Culture, Ambassadors, and PridehouseTO Celebrates! (PridehouseTO, 2015b). Through these projects, not only did the initiative continue to pursue the objectives of the inaugural Pride Houses, but also to elaborate on them substantially. Indeed, described as a province-wide initiative, PridehouseTO undertook several activities to raise awareness, generate discussions, and evoke change across the province. Notably, the organization trained two cohorts of Inclusion Ambassadors who were intended to return to their home communities to host workshops and remote Pride Houses both within and outside of the Games footprint.

Further, a partnership with the Elementary Teachers Federation of Ontario allowed for the development of an educational resource, *The Pridehouse that Kids Built* (PridehouseTO, 2015c), that was used throughout the province to support teachers in discussions of inclusion in the context of sport for elementary students in the public school systems. Further, the physical products of using this resource were then returned to Toronto and used as an art installation during the games. While PridehouseTO continued to provide the welcoming spaces, resources, and support of its predecessor, it also incorporated a variety of attempts to leverage the games to generate discussion, raise awareness, and ideally elicit broader social change in communities around the province.[6] Further, given the existing support structures in place (notably Pride House International), PridehouseTO initiatives should have benefitted substantially through the resources afforded through this network (e.g., knowledge-sharing with Pride House organizers at LEAP Sports in Glasgow and international media exposure). PridehouseTO was also the first Pride House to be included on the official cultural program of its respective games and consequently enjoyed the perks (and presumably pitfalls) of being officially recognized by the organizing committee. Not surprisingly, given the structures and resources available, we can expect that the reach and potency of the message emanating from PridehouseTO to be substantial both in Canada and abroad.

REFLECTIONS ON SPORT, DIPLOMACY, AND SOFT POWER IN CANADA

In many ways, we have constructed the Pride House Movement as a cultural export from Canada to the world in the context of sport. The past decade has included many monumental breakthroughs for sexual orientation and gender identity in sport around the world, including many athletes coming out publicly and the emergence of an LGBTQ presence at large-scale international games. However, within this, we cannot ignore the importance of social and political contexts in the process of advancing sexual rights around the world. Indeed, Sochi was instrumental in many ways in highlighting the reluctance or inability of multinational organizations (such as the IOC) to proactively address issues around human rights in the context of large-scale games. However, less than a year following the Games in Sochi, the IOC voted to include the nondiscrimination against sexual orientation clause in the sixth fundamental principle of Olympism (Morton, 2014) in the Olympic Charter (IOC, 2015). Indeed, in light of Sweibel's (2009) insights into the lack of support for public diplomacy and the resulting inability of the UN to take up conversations about sexual orientation and gender identity, we might draw a parallel to the IOC. While large, multinationals are bound by the interests of their voting members, host countries, on the other hand, are offered an international platform to address (or brush aside) human rights issues. In an age of abundance of free-flowing information, this platform has the potential to be mobilized and extended across international borders to generate discussion around issues, raise awareness about issues that might otherwise be off limits, and educate people on circumstances, public policy, and human rights in countries around the world.

While the Canadian public policy context offered fertile ground for the development of the Pride House Movement, as discussed above, we cannot assume that Canadian values are so simply homogenous. Indeed, within the diverse cultural mosaic there exist many individuals, groups, organizations, and communities who would not support efforts to fully recognize the rights of LGBTQ-identified persons. With this in mind, the selection of host cities becomes a point of interest. Both Vancouver and Toronto have vibrant existing LGBTQ communities, both with distinguishable neighbourhoods (Davie Street and the Church-Wellesley Village, respectively). Within these vibrant communities, there exist many social, cultural, and economic resources that can be drawn upon (e.g., the Church-Wellesley BIA, EGALE Canada, LEGIT/Rainbow Refuge). These cities are therefore appropriate contexts for propagating social agendas. However, other regions and cities are often less fortunate. PridehouseTO addressed this disparity in their attempts to mainstream discussions about LGBTQ persons in sport through education and outreach initiatives (e.g., *The Pridehouse that Kids Built*). Therefore, in considering Pride House initiatives within the context of event leveraging, not only do events offer a platform to exercise soft power by projecting Canadian values of tolerance and diversity on an international scale, events also provide an opportunity to (re)produce these values domestically and contribute to the alignment of policy, values, and international relationships, which, as noted by Nye (2008), is essential in public diplomacy efforts.

CONCLUSION

In summary, the Pride House Movement appears to have emerged upon the platform of large, international sport events as a means of advancing sexual rights both in Canada and abroad. In the context of Canadian host cities with (relatively) strong histories of political support for LGBTQ communities, Pride Houses provide an interesting case through which to consider the use of soft power in the hosting of large-scale sport events. Furthermore, while much of the literature discussing large-scale sport events and soft power refers to national strategies (e.g., Grix & Houlihan, 2014), Pride Houses (in Canada and abroad) have emerged and developed in ways that have largely been driven and directed by organizations outside of national governments. Thus, by considering theoretical constructs of soft power and (sport) event leveraging, the Pride House Movement offers an insightful case to consider the potential of sport events to influence public diplomacy and advance the agenda of human rights in diverse inter and intranational contexts.

While these ideas suggest an exciting potential of sport events to elicit positive social change as a form of public diplomacy, these processes are far more complex and intricate than our brief discussion suggests. Indeed, as highlighted by the work of Swiebel (2009) and the Pride House initiatives described here, existing political opportunity structures are important factors in determining the effectiveness of advancing human rights in diverse contexts. The discussion in this chapter has only scratched the surface in describing the political messiness of the work undertaken and the implications of Pride House objectives. While large-scale sport events offer a platform for discussions and the highlighting of inequalities, that alone is not sufficient to improve social contexts and lived experiences in which these events take place, let alone policy realms in which initiatives such as Pride House are barred from entering. In short, leveraging strategies and soft power are part of much larger processes involved in public diplomacy and cannot be read apart from local political contexts and international relations.

In this chapter we examined the development of the Pride House Movement in Canada, and some of the implications emanating from its development into international contexts. In Canada, there is a strong and continually evolving history of progress towards a full recognition and acceptance of sexual rights for LGBTQ-identified persons. Within this context, Pride House initiatives enjoy support of many public and private resources to pursue its objectives. Internationally, the movement has also gained traction in terms of raising awareness about inequalities and human rights issues around the world. While there is much work to be done before human rights issues relating to sexual orientation and gender identity are addressed, including full recognition of human rights by large multinationals such as the UN and the IOC, initiatives such as Pride Houses may play pivotal diplomatic roles in highlighting and possibly addressing these issues. In this case, sport diplomacy in Canada has served not only to address issues at home, but also extended beyond national borders to provoke discussions and initiatives internationally. Sport events will likely continue to offer platforms upon which human rights issues can be highlighted and these events may also influence discussions about human rights in Canada and around the world.

In summary, we would like to return to another quote from former Prime Minister Pierre Trudeau. As we have discussed, sport events have a chance to both reflect on the values of a country and share these values with the world, and we propose that hosting these events may continue to offer platforms to engage in difficult and meaningful discussions about contemporary issues in Canada. Given the time-sensitive nature of events and their potential to drive social change, we look to the metaphor of paddling a canoe, and slowly progressing with each stroke or event. Trudeau aptly summarized this progress in the forward to a book on the very Canadian sport and pastime of paddling: "May every dip of your paddle lead you towards a rediscovery of yourself" (Mason, 1980, p. v).

DISCUSSION QUESTIONS

1. Explain why the socio-political context of Canada is conducive to discussing and pushing the agenda of recognizing human and sexual rights?

2. Do a quick search of the Davie (Vancouver) or Church-Wellesley (Toronto) neighborhoods. What resources within these communities might have been drawn upon in order to host successful Pride House initiatives? How might these resources contribute to effecting policy change outside of these communities?

3. Consider your local community and the mechanisms of soft power (image building, generating a platform for dialogue, trust building, and reconciliation/integration). What initiatives might a Pride House undertake in this context? Why?

4. What are some of the challenges faced by the Pride House Movement in attempting to promote sexual rights internationally (e.g., consider developing regions or regions with strong religious influence in political decision making)?

5. Choose a business, organization, or community group in the Davie or Church-Wellesley Neighborhood (using online community directories); develop a plan for a partnership or corporate social responsibility initiative that could be undertaken between this group and a Pride House. What would the intended initiative entail? What would the intended outcomes of the initiative be? How might you evaluate these outcomes?

REFERENCES

Banting, K., & Kymlicka, W. (2010). Canadian multiculturalism: Global anxieties and local debates. *British Journal of Canadian Studies, 23*, 43-72.

Birch-Jones, J. (2010). *2010 PRIDEhouse Legacy Report*. Ottawa, ON.

Brotman, S., Ryan, B., Jalbert, Y., & Rowe, B. (2002). Reclaiming space-regaining health: The health care experiences of two-spirit people in Canada. *Journal of Gay and Lesbian Social Services, 14*, 67-87.

Canadian Civil Liberties Association. (2015). *Frequently asked questions regarding change of sex designation for trans persons*. Retrieved from https://ccla.org/frequently-asked-questions-regarding-change-of-sex-designation-for-trans-persons/

Canadian Broadcasting Corporation Digital Archives (1967, December 21). *Trudeau: 'There's no place for the state in the bedrooms of the nation.'* Retrieved from http://www.cbc.ca/archives/entry/omnibus-bill-theres-no-place-for-the-state-in-the-bedrooms-of-the-nation

Canadian Broadcasting Corporation News. (2012). *Timeline: Same-sex rights in Canada*. Retrieved from http://www.cbc.ca/news/canada/timeline-same-sex-rights-in-canada-1.1147516

Chalip, L. (2006). Towards social leverage of sport events. *Journal of Sport & Tourism, 11,* 109–127. doi:10.1080/14775080601155126

Citizenship and Immigration Canada. (2015). *Changes to gender information for citizenship documentation*. Retrieved from http://www.cic.gc.ca/english/resources/tools/cit/admin/id/change-gender.asp

Cox, L. (2015, June 2). Untitled blog post. Tumbler. [Weblog]. Retrieved on November 22, 2015, from http://lavernecox.tumblr.com/post/120503412651/on-may-29-2014-the-issue-of-timemagazine

Declaration of Montreal. (2006). [Endorsed by the] International Conference on LGBT Human Rights [of the] 1st World Outgames, Montreal 2006. Retrieved from http://www.declarationof-montreal.org/

Elling, A., & Janssens, J. (2009). Sexuality as a structural principle in sport participation: Negotiating sport spaces. *International Review for the Sociology of Sport, 44,* 71-86.

Forsyth, J. & Giles, A. R. (2012). *Aboriginal peoples and sport in Canada: Historical Foundations and Contemporary Issues*. Vancouver, BC: UBC Press.

Government of Canada (1982). *The Canadian charter of rights and freedoms*. Retrieved from http://laws-lois.justice.gc.ca/eng/const/page-15.html

Government of Canada (1985). *The Indian act*. Ottawa, ON. Retrieved from http://laws-lois.justice.gc.ca/eng/acts/i-5/

Government of Canada (2012). *Canadian multiculturalism: An inclusive citizenship*. Ottawa, ON. Retrieved from http://www.cic.gc.ca/english/multiculturalism/citizenship.asp

Giulianotti, R. (2015). The Beijing 2008 Olympics: Examining the interrelations of China, globalization, and soft power. *European Review, 23,* 286-296.

Grix, J. (2015). *Sport Politics: An Introduction*. Palgrave Macmillan.

Grix, J., (Ed.) (2014). *Leveraging legacies from sports mega-events: Concepts and cases*. London, UK: Palgrave Macmillan.

Grix, J., & Houlihan, B. (2014). Sport mega-events as part of a nation's soft power strategy: The cases of Germany (2006) and the UK (2012). *British Journal of Politics and International Relations, 16,* 572-596.

Health Canada. (2010). *Canada's Health Care System* (Medicare). Retrieved from http://www.hc-sc.gc.ca/hcs-sss/medi-assur/index-eng.php

Indigenous and Northern Affairs Canada. (2014). *Aboriginal history in Canada*. Retrieved from https://www.aadnc-aandc.gc.ca/eng/1100100013778/1100100013779

International Olympic Committee. (2015). *Olympic charter*. Lausanne, Switzerland: International Olympic Committee. Retrieved from http://www.olympic.org/olympic-charter/documents-reports-studies-publications

Jackson, S. J. (1998). Life in the (mediated) faust lane: Ben Johnson, national affect and the 1988 crisis of Canadian Identity. *International Review for the Sociology of Sport, 33,* 227-238.

Kitching, H. (2010, February 20). Olympic Pride House: Government throws a party for the gays... and the Olympic president lets the crowd know he's one of us. OutQ News. Retrieved from http://outqnews.wordpress.com/2010/02/20/olympic-pride-house-government-throws-a-party-for-the-gays/

Leslie, K. (2015, November 6). Ontario to expand medical referrals for sex-reassignment surgery. *Globe and Mail*. Retrieved from http://www.theglobeandmail.com/news/national/ontario-to-expand-medical-referrals-for-sex-reassignment-surgery/article27146437/

Mason, B. (1980). *Path of the Paddle: An Illustrated Guide to the Art of Canoeing*. Toronto, ON: Van Nostrand Reinhold

Mendelsohn, M. (2002). *Canadians thoughts on their health care system: Preserving the Canadian model through innovation*. Ottawa, ON: Commission on the Future of Health Care in Canada. Retrieved from http://www.queensu.ca/cora/_files/MendelsohnEnglish.pdf

Misener, L., McGillivray, D., McPherson, G., & Legg, D. (2015). Leveraging parasport events for sustainable community participation: The Glasgow 2014 Commonwealth Games. *Annals of Leisure Research, 18*(4), 450-469.

Misener, L. (2015). Leveraging parasport events for community participation: development of a theoretical framework. *European Sport Management Quarterly, 15*, 1–22. doi:10.1080/16184742.2014.997773

Misener, L., & Schulenkorf, N. (2016). Rethinking the social value of sport events through an asset-based community development (ABCD) perspective. *Journal of Sport Management, 30*, 329-340. doi:http://dx.doi.org/10.1123/jsm.2015-0203

Morton, B. (2014, November 19). IOC's sexual orientation clause 'exactly what they promised,' says Vancouver Coun. Tim Stevenson. *Vancouver Sun*. Retrieved from http://www.vancouversun.com/life/sexual+orientation+clause+exactly+what+they+promised+says+Vancouver+Coun+Stevenson/10393037/story.html

Nye, J. S. (2008). Public diplomacy and soft power. *Annals of the American Academy of Poitical and Social Science, 616*, 94-109.

Nygård, H. M., & Gates, S. (2013). Soft power at home and abroad: Sport diplomacy, politics and peace-building. *International Area Studies Review, 16*, 235-243.

Peesker, S. (2009, June 9). Spelling out 'LGBTTIQQ2S': A pride primer. CP24. Retrieved from http://www.cp24.com/spelling-out-lgbttiqq2s-a-pride-primer-1.405889

PridehouseTO. (2015a). *About*. Retrieved from http://www.pridehouseto.ca/about/

PridehouseTO. (2015b). *Projects*. Retrieved from http://www.pridehouseto.ca/projects/

PridehouseTO. (2015c). *The Pridehouse that kids built*. Retrieved from http://www.pridehouseto.ca/projects/phtkb/

Pride House International. (2015a). *Pride house history*. Retrieved from http://www.pridehouseinternational.org/index.php/history/

Pride House International. (2015b). *2014 Sochi Olympics, remote*. Retrieved from http://www.pridehouseinternational.org/index.php/2014-sochi-olympics-remote/

Pride House International. (2015c). *2015 Pan/Parapan Am Games, Toronto, Canada*. Retrieved from http://www.pridehouseinternational.org/index.php/2015-panamparapanam-games-toronto-canada/

Re:searching for LGBTQ Health. (2015). *Two-spirit community*. Toronto, ON: University of Toronto & The Canadian Association for Mental Health. Retrieved from http://lgbtqhealth.ca/community/two-spirit.php

Rothman, S. B. (2011). Revising the soft power concept: What are the means and mechanisms of soft power? *Journal of Political Power, 4*, 49-64.

Schulenkorf, N. (2010). The roles and responsibilities of a change agent in sport event development projects. *Sport Management Review, 13*, 118–128. doi:10.1016/j.smr.2009.05.001

Smith, M. (1999). *Lesbian and gay rights in Canada: Social movements and equality seeking, 1971 - 1995*. Toronto, ON: University of Toronto Press.

Strapagiel, L. (2015, April 28). Transgender Canadians can now self-identify on citizenship documents without sex-reassignment surgery. *National Post*. Retrieved from http://news.nationalpost.com/news/canada/federal-government-quietly-eases-requirements-for-canadians-seeking-to-change-gender-on-citizen-certificate

Swiebel, J. (2009). Lesbian, gay, bisexual and transgender human rights: The search for an international strategy. *Contemporary Politics, 15*, 19-35.

Taks, M., Green, B. C., Misener, L., & Chalip, L. (2014). Evaluating sport development outcomes: the case of a medium-sized international sport event. *European Sport Management Quarterly, 14*, 213–237. doi:10.1080/16184742.2014.882370

Truth and Reconciliation Commission of Canada. (2015). *TRC findings*. Winnipeg, MB: Truth and Reconciliation Commission of Canada. Retrieved from http://www.trc.ca/websites/trcinstitution/index.php?p=890

Vance, J. F. (2009). *A history of Canadian culture: From petroglyphs to product, circuses to the CBC.* Don Mills, ON: Oxford University Press.

Wilson, B. (2006). Selective memory in a global culture: Reconsidering links between youth, hockey, and Canadian identity. In D. Whitson & R. Gruneau (Eds.), *Artificial Ice: Hockey, Culture, and Commerce,* (pp. 52-70). Peterborough, ON: Garamond Press.

Yogyakarta Principles [on the Application of International Human Rights Law in Relation to Sexual Orientation and Gender Identity]. (2007). Retrieved from http://www.yogyakartaprinciples.org/

You Can Play. (n.d.). *Our cause.* Retrieved from http://youcanplayproject.org/pages/our-cause

ENDNOTES

[1]   It should be acknowledged that we use this term as it is customary in the literature as well in the Pridehouse documentation. The acronym, however, does not come without tensions, and as a result, is sometimes expanded to included many other categories (e.g., LGBTTIQQ2S: lesbian, gay, bisexual, transgender, transsexual, intersex, queer, questioning, and 2 spirited, see Peesker, 2009). As noted by Swiebel (2009) the focus on binaries (e.g., man/woman, homo/heterosexual) may serve to (re)produce the very power structures that much of the human rights movement seeks to address. Alternatively, we may use the term *queer* as all-encompassing, or shift the focus to *sexual orientation and gender identity* (SOGI) or *sexual rights,* both of which have been adopted in some contexts. Throughout this paper, these terminologies (*LGBTQ, queer,* and *SOGI*) are used interchangeably.

[2]   First coined at the Third Annual Inter-tribal Native American, First Nations, Gay and Lesbian American Conference in Winnipeg in 1990, this term is used by First Nations people. The term is sacred, describing someone who has both masculine and feminine spirits, and does not exclusively refer to sexual attraction or gender roles (Re:searching for LGBTQ Health, 2015). As we do not take up the politics of colonialism in this chapter, we do not address the many additional implications of public policy for indigenous and two-spirited peoples. For a more detailed discussion, see Brotman, Ryan, Jalbert, and Rowe (2002).

[3]   We use this vernacular as it is currently used by Pride House International. Since 2010, Pride House organizations have used different vernacular, including PRIDE house and Pridehouse.

[4]   While we cannot hope to do this topic justice in such a short section, we hope that this brief summary might provide some insight into some political issues and events that have shaped political realities of indigenous peoples in Canada. For insight into historical and contemporary perspectives on Aboriginal peoples and sport in Canada, see Forsyth and Giles (2012).

[5]   Also see this reference for a much more detailed timeline of events related to same-sex rights and policy in Canada. The CBC also has an excellent archive of media coverage of many major political developments in Canada.

[6]   It should be noted that, at the time of writing, final reports from PridehouseTO are still not available. However, as more information becomes available, it will be accessible on the Pride House International website (Pride House International, 2015c).

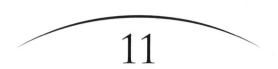

11

SOUTH SUDAN'S QUEST FOR INTERNATIONAL ACCEPTANCE AND INTERNAL IDENTITY THROUGH SPORT: "WE ARE GOING TO TAKE CARE OF HER LIKE A DAUGHTER"

MYLES SCHRAG

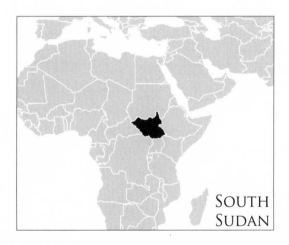

SOUTH
SUDAN

At its 128th session on Sunday, August 2, 2015, the International Olympic Committee (IOC) officially and unanimously recognized South Sudan as its 206th member. An undeniable atmosphere of hope filled the Kuala Lumpur (Malaysia) Convention Centre. The upbeat news belied all the difficulty it took to get the world's newest country to that moment, and more importantly, all the uncertainty still engulfing South Sudan.

Though southern Sudan had been at war with Sudan for decades and South Sudan had been at war with itself for two years, on this day Sudanese sporting officials were there in a show of support, and the IOC praised them for helping South Sudan in its Olympic quest.

"All the sports facilities are broken down," said South Sudan national Olympic committee president Wilson Deng Kuoirot, who himself broke down in tears at one point. "Most of the children now have joined the armed groups. We are going to arm them with sports instead of with guns. . . . I am delighted and exhilarated. This will promote reconciliation and national unity." ("South Sudan to Compete in Rio," 2015).

It was understood that international aid would be needed to help build up South Sudan's sporting infrastructure. IOC president, Thomas Bach, acknowledged as much when he said,

> Let me wish you a very bright future. We will stand by your side. We look
> forward to welcoming you to the opening ceremony of the Olympic Games
> of Rio de Janeiro [in 2016]. This will put your nation on the world map.
> (Grohmann, 2015)

Technically speaking, South Sudan joined the world map as an independent country on July 9, 2011, and a United Nations member five days later. But Bach's words are worth examining with a pragmatic lens. The speeches in Malaysia were overwhelmingly positive and uplifting, about the country of South Sudan, which drifted into civil war since voting for its independence; about the power of sport; and about the power of the Olympic Movement. It is clear that the sports officials in South Sudan want to use sport to figuratively put their nation on the world map, a common tool that countries employ as an alternative to more explicit forms of diplomacy (Dichter, 2014).

Step away from that historic day, though, and reality sets in. Any new nation will experience growing pains. Here is a country ravaged by decades of war that spurred separation from its neighbor to the north, and it is now depleted even further because of sectarian fighting and alleged human rights abuses from both its government and rebel forces. Just the fact that it took more than four years to gain the required five approved national sport federations needed for IOC membership is an indication of how difficult the young country is finding it to prioritize sport in any substantial way.

Officially making it possible that August day for eligible athletes to compete at the 2016 Rio Games was just the beginning, and despite the long road it took to get there, that was perhaps the easiest part of South Sudan's diplomatic efforts involving sport. As this chapter will show, the country's strategy for using sport and diplomacy is still evolving. Scholarly literature on South Sudan's sporting initiatives is therefore understandably limited. Unlike countries with more stability and history, we will explore South Sudan's development almost literally from the ground up. In the absence of policies either clearly implemented or having had the chance to be completed, we will examine what direction the nation's sport leaders could or should go. The 2016 Rio Games are now closed. The Olympiad exposed shortcomings by the young country's national Olympic committee (NOC), and highlighted just how many critical questions face South Sudan's sporting future.

UNDERSTANDING THE STATE OF SOUTH SUDAN

Though the situation in South Sudan will likely remain volatile for some time, a brief discussion of its geopolitical and economic status, as well as its sporting context, will provide helpful background for the miniature SWOT (strengths, weaknesses, opportunities, and threats) analysis and recommendations for the country later in the chapter. See Figure 1 for a timeline of key events in South Sudan's history in and out of sport.

✳ Figure 11-1. Timeline of Key Events in South Sudan History ✳

1955	First Sudanese Civil War begins.
1956	Sudan becomes an independent country despite tensions.
1972	First Sudanese Civil War ends.
1983	Start of the Second Sudanese Civil War; amateur basketball player Manute Bol leaves country before hostilities commence.
2005	Comprehensive Peace Agreement ends Second Civil War.
2008	Lost Boy and American citizen Lopez Lomong carries U.S. flag during Opening Ceremony of Beijing Olympics.
2010	Manute Bol dies of liver failure.
2011	South Sudan votes to become an independent country with over 98% in favor. Independence day occurs July 9. Fighting over contested oil-rich states in Sudan commences between Sudan and South Sudan.
2012	South Sudan joins FIFA and plays first national soccer game; Lost Boy Guor Marial runs in Olympic marathon as an "Independent Olympic Athlete." Luol Deng becomes NBA All-Star for Chicago Bulls.
2013	South Sudan Civil War erupts. Marial gains U.S. citizenship and visits South Sudan for first time in 20 years.
2015	Margrat Rumat Hassan runs 400m at Youth Olympic Games.
2016	Ousted vice president Riek Machar, a Nuer, returns to office under President Salva Kiir, a Dinka, as part of a power-sharing agreement. Further violence ensues. Guor Miading Miaker is country's first Olympic flag-bearer, leading three-athlete delegation. Thon Maker was drafted in the first round by the NBA Milwaukee Bucks. Maker was born in the city of Wau in what is now South Sudan.

GEOPOLITICAL AND ECONOMIC STATUS

Fighting between predominantly Islamic, Arabic northern Sudan and indigenously African, increasingly Christian southern Sudan began even before Sudan gained its independence in 1956 and has continued with few interruptions ever since. Deng (2001) described the extent of the conflict:

> This war has raged intermittently since 1955, making it possibly the longest civil conflict in the world. It continues unabated, mostly outside the focus of diplomacy or the attention of international media, taking a huge and terrible human toll. Over two million people have died as a result of the war and

related causes, such as war-induced famine. About five million people have been displaced, while half a million more have fled across an international border. Tens of thousands of women and children have been abducted and subjected to slavery. By all accounts, it appears to be the worst humanitarian disaster in the world today."

The Comprehensive Peace Agreement (CPA) was signed in 2005 by the Sudan People's Liberation Movement from the south and the government of Sudan, whose capital is Khartoum in the north. The CPA led to an autonomous government in southern Sudan and eventual independence in 2011. During this period, tensions remained high between the north and south.

With independence approaching in July 2011, the contested Sudanese states of South Kordofan and Blue Nile became the source of renewed fighting between Sudan and South Sudan. The regions, which most notably include oil-rich Abyei Area, include many sympathetic to South Sudan, and the fighting has continued in what has been called Sudan's "third civil war" (Edun, 2011). Conflict turned inward among various nomadic groups in South Sudan after the official split from Sudan because of a lethal mix of cattle rustling and heavily armed ethnic militias. The most lethal period began in December 2013, as rebels led by ousted vice president Riek Machar, a Nuer, and government forces under President Salva Kiir, a Dinka, resulted in tens of thousands being killed and more than 2.2 million being displaced (Grohmann 2015). The Dinkas are the largest and the Nuers are the second largest among dozens of ethnic groups in South Sudan ("South Sudan rebel Riek Machar," 2013).

As part of a power-sharing agreement, Machar was sworn in as vice president in a tense ceremony on April 26, 2016. Much trepidation accompanied this latest twist, as previous cease-fires from almost two years of peace negotiations had been repeatedly broken. UN peacekeepers continued to shelter tens of thousands of displaced people, Juba remained militarized, and Kiir's plan to divide South Sudan's 10 states into 28 and appoint governors in those all left the young country in a state of confusion (Fortin, 2016).

South Sudan relies heavily on a relatively large oil supply for its economy. Given the decades of war, the young nation's ability to leverage any of its resources, including its population, has been sorely compromised. This is the environment in which Kuoirot and sports leaders want to create an infrastructure that can help the country gain international acceptance and develop high-level athletes and a respected sporting culture.

SPORTING CONTEXT

Just days before Machar's return to Juba—in fact, as his return was being delayed due to last-minute negotiations about how many rebel soldiers would be allowed to accompany him and what the public ceremony would look like—the national stadium played host to a Wrestling for Peace competition in which the top prize was five cattle. The event, backed by the U.S. governmental aid agency USAID, was the first in the capital since a wrestling tournament in December 2013 was interrupted by factional fighting. The mood, according to spectators quoted at the venue, was encouraging as it related to sport and subdued as it related to the country's future. One T-shirt read, "Wrestling for peace, forgiveness and reconciliation" (De Souza, 2016). Said Philip Jok, a Dinka tribesman, "Wrestling is not going to stop the war. But getting together like this, well, we can see we don't have to fight each other" (De Souza, 2016). And from tournament organizer Peter Biar Ajak, a refugee who returned home as a Harvard-trained economist, "The war has to end and life goes on. This is a way of saying we want peace" (De Souza, 2016).

Though wrestling is a popular traditional pastime across tribal lines in South Sudan, the modern sporting world is essential to attracting attention beyond the new country's borders. In order to be admitted into the IOC, South Sudan needed to have at least five sports federations officially recognized by international governing bodies. An NOC was only formed two months before the IOC session in Malaysia, but South Sudan had seven federations in place and either accepted or provisionally accepted by the time of the IOC vote. Those were, according to Edward SeTimo, secretary general for sports at the Ministry of Culture, Youth and Sport, soccer, basketball, athletics (track and field), table tennis, handball, judo, and taekwondo. South Sudan joined the Fédération Internationale de Football Association (FIFA) in 2012 and played its first international soccer game on July 10, 2012, one year and one day after its independence. The soccer team failed to qualify for the 2018 Men's World Cup. South Sudan joined two other powerful organizations, the International Basketball Federation (FIBA) in 2013 and the International Association of Athletics Federations (IAAF) in 2014.

"RUNNER WITHOUT A COUNTRY"

South Sudan's inability to organize its NOC shortly after its independence led to surprising international attention leading up to the 2012 London Olympics. The plight of the young country seemed embodied in one young athlete. Guor Marial, one of the so-called "Lost Boys of Sudan," who was displaced during the Second Civil War period between 1983 and 2005, qualified for the marathon. Marial had fled his village in southern Sudan in 1993 and eventually was granted residence in the United States, attending Iowa State University. Marial could not run for the new country of South Sudan at the London Games because it didn't have an NOC. He refused to run under Sudan's flag because of the atrocities committed against his family and friends in the war, including the death of 28 family members, eight of whom were siblings. The IOC allowed him to compete under the Olympic flag, wearing a singlet with the acronym IOA (Independent Olympic Athlete), becoming the first person to do so (Wade, 2014). This led to Marial being dubbed "the runner without a country." He had many opportunities to talk about his own story and the story of his homeland before and after his 47th place finish in the race—a race he didn't know if he would be allowed to run until only a week before the Olympics. He remains the face of South Sudan in many news accounts about the country's sports scene. Marial, now Guor Miading Miaker, trained in Kenya leading up to the 2016 Summer Games. He watched the IOC vote on the Internet from Kenya and told the Associated Press

> This moment is so special for me and my country, and it will be next year when I walk into the stadium in Rio behind our own flag. We can bring unity, and the sport we have initiated across the country can unite all 64 tribes and all 10 states. ("South Sudan to Compete in Rio," 2015)

When I spoke to Marial in early 2013, the runner clearly was still making sense of all the publicity from the previous eight months. Extremely friendly, relaxed, and appreciative of all the support he had received, he did not know what his next steps as an athlete would be. He spoke of being "passionate" that sport is a unifier, especially for the youth in South Sudan. He wanted to explore ideas for how to do that. At the same time, he acknowledged the logistical difficulty of being in contact with the sports ministry, the lack of funding for the sports ministry, and his plans to return to his home region for the first time in 20 years later that summer. Then, he said, he could get a better idea of what needed to be done.

"You just take it a little bit at a time," Marial said. "If you think about it, you stress. There's either an answer or no answer. And you go from there" (personal communication, March 29, 2013).

Guor Miading Miaker has been busy since the London Olympics. A documentary about him, called "Runner without a Country," had filmmaker Bill Gallagher following him around the world. Miading Miaker set up training camp in Kenya, and invited promising South Sudanese runners to join him. He became a U.S. citizen in February 2013, which gave him dual citizenship, and having a U.S. passport allowed him to return to South Sudan for the first time in 20 years to visit family. "Now, two countries are my country," he quipped (Gambaccini, 2013). Miading Miaker believes that the best move he can make for South Sudan is to run well as a representative of his country. He could run for either the United States or South Sudan, but after a period of time where he was noncommittal about which country he would seek to represent, he chose South Sudan:

> The decision to represent South Sudan won because of the great need for peace and stability by me and by my people in South Sudan. We have been in a long life of suffering, and we have lost millions of lives due to civil war. Majority of the generations before me, my generation, and the generations after me have never had childhood experience because of war. As the son and a citizen of South Sudan, I strongly felt that I must bring my athletic skills to South Sudan to help build peace in the country . . . . I feel as a citizen of the South Sudan and the US, it's my responsibility to turn this negative for a positive by promoting peace through sports. I want to give hope to refugees, stateless, and homeless around the world that there is a tomorrow. Don't give in on a dark day because the greatness is yet to come. Work hard, believe

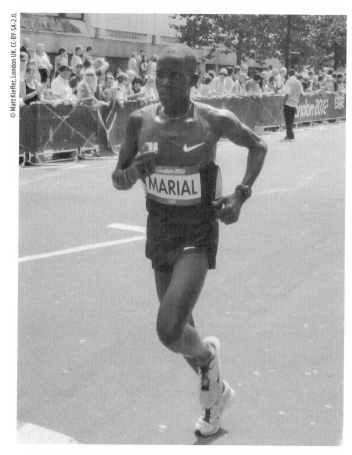

Guor Miading Miaker competing in the London Summer Olympics, 2012.

in yourself, have a faith, be positive about life, and know that there are kind people out there thinking about you. (Wade, 2014)

OTHER ATHLETES FROM SOUTH SUDAN

Despite the political unrest of the past three decades, a number of athletes originally from southern Sudan have gained international acclaim, most prominently in basketball. Indeed, in my 2013 conversation with Marial, he stressed how much athletic talent there was in South Sudan if there were the stability in the country to cultivate it (personal communication, March 29, 2013). Currently, the fledgling nation does not have an international standard track and just one basketball stadium in the capital of Juba that 10 teams share ("South Sudan to compete in Rio," 2015).

The most prominent basketball player from southern Sudan was Manute Bol, one of the tallest and most prolific shot blockers in the history of the National Basketball Association (NBA). He left Sudan in 1983, just before the Second Civil War broke out. His playing career and post-basketball life were marked by tireless activism on the part of refugees and reconciliation efforts between Sudan and southern Sudan before he died of kidney failure in 2010, 13 months before South Sudan's birth.

Other basketball players from southern Sudan include Luol Deng, whose family escaped Sudan when he was a child and has since become a two-time All-Star for the Chicago Bulls; Kueth Duany, captain of the 2003 Syracuse national championship team; Deng Gai, who played briefly with the Philadelphia 76ers and is a cousin of Luol Deng; and Ater Majok, who played at the University of Connecticut and professionally in eight countries.

Deng and Bol, both Dinkas, met in Egypt after Deng's family had fled Sudan. Deng eventually settled in London and became a British citizen, playing for England's national team in the Olympics. The Luol Deng Foundation has been active in South Sudan, starting a basketball camp there in 2011, and Deng himself traveled to Juba when independence was announced. When an outdoor court in Bol's honor was dedicated in 2015, Deng posted on social media through Instagram:

> Manute Bol Court was officially opened on August 6, 2015, in Juba, South Sudan. On the list of accomplished I've been blessed to achieve, this is very high on my list as one of the most memorable ones. The faces of smiling youth made it an instant success in my book. Thank you to everyone who made this possible #SouthSudanUnite #OnePeople. (Collins, 2015)

Like Miading Miaker, others see South Sudan's athletic potential in its youth. "You know, if you draw a basketball player you draw a Sudanese or a Dinka and that's exciting because they are tall, they're coordinated, they're athletic, and that's what the game of basketball needs," Deng said. "There's a lot of talent and raw ability," agreed Patrick Engelbrecht, a coach with NBA Africa, the league's development arm, who joined Deng in Juba on South Sudan's independence day. "They are blessed with the right physical attributes: their height, coordination, fluidity, their sheer size. The challenge is helping local coaches cultivate that talent" (McConnell, 2011).

In track and field, Lopez Lomong is a two-time Olympian for the United States after becoming an American citizen. He was chosen by his teammates to be the flag bearer at the opening ceremony for the 2008 Beijing Games. Like Miading Miaker, Lomong was a "Lost Boy," taken from his family at a church service by soldiers at age 6. He spent 10 years at a refugee camp in Kenya before being adopted by an American family in 2001, shortly before the 9/11 terrorist attacks shuttered the refugee relocation program. Lomong has actively provided relief in the form of schools and clean water in his native country (Lomong, 2012).

A 16 year old gave South Sudan a female track star to root for on the international stage when Margrat Rumat Hassan ran the 400 meters at the 2015 Youth Olympics in Nanjing, China. When the IOC granted South Sudan membership, Hassan was the other individual athlete, along with Miading Miaker, who was prominently mentioned as being assured of having a country to represent in Rio. As we will discover in the Weaknesses section later in this chapter, Hassan and Miading Miaker only were able to wear their country's uniform in Rio after some last-minute controversy.

"We have nothing, we are starting from scratch," said Tong Deran, South Sudan Olympic committee secretary general. He explained that he hoped the committee would empower young athletes like Hassan. "We are going to take care of her like a daughter" ("South Sudan to Compete in Rio," 2015).

Given the monumental challenges of the country, Deran's paternal instincts will be a tough order to fulfill. Can the sporting establishment support its athletes in preparing them to perform? And can sport live up to the promise that so many claim is possible in helping South Sudan prosper?

WHAT DOES SPORT DIPLOMACY MEAN FOR SOUTH SUDAN?

Governments typically intervene in international sport for three primary reasons:

- to maintain and strengthen alliances,
- to promote policies or political positions at home and abroad, and
- to increase national prestige.

Further, "States created as a result of decolonization after World War II used sport as a way to gain recognition or international prominence, or they sought to use sport as a way to promote their political agendas through public diplomacy" (Dichter, 2014). South Sudan's moment of independence came decades after many of those states, and it stemmed from a deep rift with its tenuous neighbor in northern Sudan that served as a de facto tyrant in South Sudan's eyes just as oppressive as the European colonial powers. But South Sudan saw the importance of sport in a similar fashion. On July 21, 2011, after the creation of South Sudan, Xan Rice wrote in *The Guardian,* "A new country needs many things: passports, stamps, a currency, an international dialing code, to name a few. For Republic of South Sudan, there was a further urgent priority—"a football team" (Dichter, 2014). The South Sudan national soccer team played its first match, a 3-1 loss to a Kenyan Premier League team during independence celebrations in July 2011, and joined the Confederation of African Football (CAF) and FIFA within a year. Sport, it seems, has as much cache as stamps.

Understanding the interface between sport and diplomacy has always been a slippery proposition. The chapters in this book simultaneously reinforce Murray's criticism of sport diplomacy scholarship and practice—anecdotal, sporadic, case-specific—and provide an antidote to what he says is needed—further debate between theorists and practitioners of both diplomacy and sport (Murray, 2012). Similarly, despite the growth of sport for development and peace (SDP) scholarship and practice in the past 15 years, great skepticism accompanies discussions about what SDP's actual contributions are. SDP can be construed so broadly as to be considered meaningless, a vague and weakly theorized banner (Coalter, 2010) that is sometimes criticized for being run by pollyannish functionalists, not tying into more established development literature, and not conducting sufficient research into the efficacy of SDP programs. Diplomacy and development are certainly not interchangeable terms, though the latter can often be in the service of the former. They are linked here simply to show how sport's involvement in both cases can be used to express whatever end of the spectrum a researcher or a practitioner wishes". Sport is either a low-risk component of a public diplomacy strategy to positively affect another region of the world that has strategic value (in the case of diplomacy) or can provide assistance (in the case of development). Alternatively, sport is a tepid, politically safe tool that can appear to be more successful than it actually is, whether toward diplomatic ends or a developmental legacy.

Attempting to reconcile these two extremes raises an important question asked by Murray: Do the benefits outweigh the dangers of mixing sport and diplomacy (Murray, 2012)? At least in most cases of sport diplomacy, one can point to the successes and failures of a sport-centered policy over a period of time and comfortably assert the impact of sport. At this point in time, that is difficult to do for South Sudan. Necessarily, this chapter is more concerned with how the young nation is developing from the ground up, not rebooting or strategizing for specific geopolitical aims, e.g., the United States or Soviet Union during the Cold War. A useful approach is to temper the well-established label *public diplomacy,* under which *sport diplomacy* usually resides, and consider South Sudan's task at hand as a nation-branding initiative. Public diplomacy traditionally means government communication aimed at foreign audiences to achieve changes in the hearts and minds of the people (Szondi, 2008).

Nation branding, though practiced for decades, has only appeared in the scholarly literature since the 1990s. "Nation branding concerns applying branding and marketing communications techniques to promote a nation's image" (Fan, 2006), with the government as the initiator of branding (Gudjonsson, 2005). Public diplomacy and nation branding are sometimes intertwined, and the distinction between them is often confused in the literature. Here, we refer to nation branding as relying on communication and marketing skills, often through subtle means, resulting in a more positive view of the initiating country. Public diplomacy, often born in times of crisis, pushes for new attitudes and assertive actions from a people toward a government (Szondi, 2008). While South Sudan remains in crisis, its lack of international influence makes public diplomacy less critical than nation branding as a sympathetic underdog with an idealistic goal of self-determination. The nature of nation branding, with its marketing emphasis on targets that can be influenced, is more realistic than the messy work of diplomacy, whose groups are often more difficult to successfully message. Sport can help South Sudan if it chooses that approach.

Consider the four propositions that Jarvie puts forward regarding the potential of sport to play a role in reconciliation, reconstruction, and resolution. He doesn't suggest sport is a panacea, especially, for example, in Darfur, Sudan. Jarvie does, however, state that sport as a form of social intervention has often been overlooked to our detriment. The four propositions (Jarvie, 2013):

1. that sport matters in world politics because it can provide opportunities for diplomatic interventions at times when other forms of international relations and mediation are not working,

2.   that sport provides a popular prism through which nation-states can and do present an image to both the rest of the world and their own people,

3.   that sport can be a facilitator of change within a country, and

4.   that historical ideals of sport being a cathartic form of war without weapons should be replaced by more progressive realist cases of sport being part of a holistic package or resources that any foreign ministry or office has at its disposal.

Though Jarvie uses the term *public diplomacy* in recommending sport as a governmental tool, when looking at his list, nation branding can arguably result from numbers 2, 3, and 4. It is not hard to view South Sudan as too beset by immediate needs and crises to craft a coherent nation-branding strategy involving sport, yet sport properly understood, strategically, can and should be a means to give the country an identity to show to the rest of the world. A SWOT analysis can help explain why sport is of real value to the country.

A SWOT ANALYSIS FOR SOUTH SUDAN

A very brief SWOT analysis will review the points already covered and present several additional examples. This will show where the young country is succeeding and where it is struggling in its diplomacy and branding efforts to guide a discussion of recommendations that South Sudan should pursue going forward.

Strengths

The IOC recognition took a long time to consummate, leaving athletes like Miading Miaker and Hassan dangling as they tried to represent the new land in international competitions between 2011 and 2015. However, accomplishing the job prior to the 2016 Rio Olympics ultimately was a success and important to setting a larger agenda into motion. It ensures South Sudan will get financial aid from the IOC to build athletic facilities, and it aligns the young nation in a visible, meaningful way with the international community.

The country is now attempting to build on that achievement. Acceptance by FIFA and the Confederation of African Football ranked almost as high as belonging to the United Nations and African Union (Dewaal, 2012). One of the nation's earliest efforts after becoming a sovereign entity was to establish cultural initiatives, including sport, to establish unity (Ylönen, 2012).

> We need to build the infrastructure and what's exciting is that even at the highest levels of government there is a willingness to invest in basketball, they realize what the game can do in teaching the children the right values but also on the global stage. (McConnell, 2011)

Said NBA Africa's vice president Amadou Gallo Fall, "With a strong reputation in basketball and athletics, and a small contingent of athletes representing and speaking about the issues of South Sudan in Rio, messaging is underway." There are other examples. Symbolically, the "Independence Half Marathon" on July 11, 2015, showed a country coming together through sport. The platform that stars such as Miading Miaker, Lomong, Deng, and Bol have used, over the past decade especially, means that South Sudan and sport have a synergy that many countries take much longer to reach.

Weaknesses

In general terms, a long civil war with Sudan and the more recent conflict within the newly constructed borders are obvious weaknesses. Specifically, it creates a decimated youth culture. Sport is often about youth, and the lost youth creates an inherent problem in making sport a priority. According to the South Sudan Centre for Census, Statistics and Evaluation in 2010, only 22% of South Sudan's rural population age 15 and above can read and write, and 68% have never attended school (Boboya, 2015). Violence had subsided in Juba as Machar made his return in April 2016. Yet fighting continued around the country, food prices had reached record highs, and inflation was soaring, according to a report from the UN Food and Agriculture Organization: "Alarming reports of starvation, acute malnutrition and catastrophe levels of food insecurity have been reported in areas worst affected by the ongoing violence," the FAO report said at the time (De Souza, 2016).

There are mixed messages about how these problems might be addressed. Five key thematic issues were identified as priority areas for post-conflict state-building and peace-building in South Sudan:

1. resolving border-related disputes;
2. peace-building and reconciliation among the various ethnic communities;
3. promoting security sector reform and democratization;
4. providing development infrastructure and social amenities; and
5. creating employment, especially for youth.

Further, responses by South Sudanese stakeholders were largely consistent with priority areas that government policymakers have stated (Omeje, 2014). Sport could arguably play a role in three of these (2, 4, and 5). However, in a 2,000-word Policy Strategy Paper on Youth Employment Creation and Income Generation in South Sudan, there is not a single mention of sport (2014). While sport is mentioned in Boboya's report (2015) as a priority to engaging people across ethnic lines, he also notes that the Minister of Youth and Sport did not create a mechanism for a youth-governing body that can address issues of concern identified by youth themselves.

A sign of the weakness in the national sporting leadership emerged early in 2015 with a dispute involving marathoner Miading Miaker. The runner said that the South Sudan Athletic Federation secretary-general, Kamal John Akol, asked him to hand over funds that he received from the IOC. The secretary-general maintained that the federation's policy was to administer funds rather than have money going directly to the athletes. Miading Miaker countered that it was a scholarship for training from the IOC. Because he didn't abide Akol's request, South Sudan's marathoning ambassador from the 2012 Olympics was suspended. While the incident was quickly resolved and the runner reinstated, with him reaffirming his wish to represent South Sudan, the negative attention internationally was a shift in a story that had only been positive up to that point.

On the eve of the Rio Games, Miading Miaker and Hassan had not met the Olympic qualifying standard. In some awkward maneuvering by South Sudan's NOC, they still became two of the three track athletes that represented the country. When the South Sudan Athletics Federation was allowed two open spots, they chose Mangar Makur Chuot, a former refugee living in Australia who was the national 200-meter champion, and Santino Kenyi, the national 1500-meter record holder. The National Olympic Committee overruled the national governing body, and uninvited Chuot in favor of Hassan, who was not the country's fastest woman sprinter. The NOC secretary-general, Tong Chor Malek Deran, stated clearly that he felt pressure to choose Hassan because she was featured in a Samsung commercial entering the Olympic stadium with her fellow South Sudanese chanting her name in a sign of unity (Doherty, 2016). Miading Miaker was allowed to compete by the IOC and the IAAF under unclear circumstances, other than that he embodied the Olympic spirit. The marathoner explained in a confusing Facebook post on August 22, 2016:

> To my fellow South Sudanese athletes, I want to take this opportunity to clarify to you of my appointing to participate in this Olympic. I've seen that some of you are very disappointed for being left out of the team and have wrote complains, which I completely understand. But I want to let you know that I was not selected by the South Sudan Athletic Federation or by the South Sudan National Olympic Committee. I was given exception by the IAAF and the IOC because of my previous participation in the 2012 Olympic. As some of you may have read or heard, I was not part of the team! So South Sudan Athletic Federation and its NOC has nothing to do with my participation in this Olympic. Please don't feel so betrayed because I came and you didn't. Also, we all have to realize that none of us made a qualifying time for the Olympic. And without qualifying time, our case against the athletic federation is meaningless. Yes, there was indeed unfair selection on women side, but we have no power when we don't have qualified times. What we all need to do going forward is focus on achieving qualify standard for next international events. And if South Sudan Athletic Federation left us out of the team after that, then we will have strong case to fight for. Also, we must understand the IAAF and the IOC selection rules. That will helps us much as on how to deal with the federation. Please don't lose your hope or dream of representing South Sudan or your second nation if you wish to do so. My great wishes to all of you on your trainings.

The whole situation created a public relations fiasco that calls into question who influences national team selection, which only hurts a country's opportunity to use sport for positive publicity.

Opportunities

Despite the decimation of youth because of the Lost Boy years and ongoing fighting, a study shows that significant numbers of displaced youth have been returning to the capital city of Juba in recent years with a desire to reintegrate into the society they fled (Ensor, 2013). South Sudan has several hundred language groups, making it one of the most linguistically diverse countries on the continent (Rice, 2011). That is a challenge for communication, but the variety also means that the physical activity of sport becomes an ideal context to help unify the country under the official language of English. Team sports such as basketball and soccer, and individual sports such as athletics, offer tremendous opportunities for South Sudan, as do the corresponding attention that star athletes in those sports have garnered for the country's citizens. The foundations of Deng and Lomong provide examples of tangible infrastructure support both in and out of sport. The words and deeds by these athletes on and off the playing fields also provide significant opportunity to create a foundation on which to build international understanding about South Sudan.

Powerful organizations, including the UN, the IOC, FIFA, FIBA, and professional sports leagues, have long recognized the importance of contributing to strife-ridden regions of the world. The UN, the only organization on that list without a vested interest in sport, has declared April 6 the International Day of Sport for Development and Peace and has an International Working Group that supports ways for sport to achieve the Millennium Development Goals. The other entities, for multiple reasons, occasionally speak out about politics and violence, which can influence opinion and raise awareness about countries in turmoil and transition such as South Sudan. Early in 2016, the IOC announced the creation of Team Refugee Olympic Athletes, which resulted in an Olympic squad in Rio of 10 members from a pool of 43, five of whom were South Sudanese runners. This measure, funded by Olympic Solidarity, stemmed in large part from the Syrian refugee crisis of 2015-16, though the presentation of the initiative clearly intended for an all-inclusive approach to understanding the plight of refugees. One can surmise that the attention Marial received in 2012 also prompted the IOC to take action. The official press release from March 2, 2016, stated,

> The IOC already works with a number of United Nations agencies to help refugees around the world. For the last 20 years, the IOC and UNHCR [United Nations High Commissioner for Refugees] in particular have been using sport to support healing and development among young refugees in many camps and settlements around the world. They have consequently seen thousands of refugees benefit from sports programmes and equipment donated by the IOC." (International Olympic Committee, 2016)

Such initiatives provide opportunities for South Sudan to gain a greater understanding from the world community, if the country's sporting establishment is able to capitalize on them.

Threats

News stories that show the damage and desperation of southern Sudan's history through a sporting lens create an opportunity for education as well. But they also create a threat to positive messaging that South Sudan needs to thrive. When Jonathan Nicola was arrested April 15, 2016, in Windsor, Ontario, Canada, this tension between opportunity and threat became apparent. Nicola was playing for a high school basketball team in Canada, when it was discovered that he had previously applied to enter the United States as a refugee. Those documents showed he was born in 1986, making him 29 years old when he was playing against teenagers. Not surprisingly, Deng was called upon for comment. Deng didn't defend the ruse, but he cautioned against judgment of Nicola and said not to assume he was doing it for sport-centered reasons. "There's a lot of things—not just in the South Sudan, but all over the world—there's a lot of things going on," Deng said.

People are going to do whatever it takes just to have a better life. Sometimes it might not be what we agree with, and it's not the right thing but until you hear his side of the story, you don't really know what's going on. (Duff, 2016)

With reasoned voices like Deng's, a threat becomes an opportunity.

Back in South Sudan, the strife between government and rebel factions is well-documented, and its ramifications cannot be underestimated, in or out of sport. It creates a culture of distrust, in-country training becomes difficult at best and, more often, a dangerous proposition. External support becomes more difficult to galvanize. Two obstacles must be overcome specific to South Sudan's sport diplomacy efforts: the social unrest and decimation of its young population, necessitating a realistic strategy about the role of sport and the changing nature of conflict (Annan & Mousavizadeh, 2012), and an inability to leverage strengths while mitigating weaknesses, which is seen most clearly in the debacle between the SSAF and Miading Miaker, and later between the NOC and Chuot.

SOUTH SUDAN, LOOKING AHEAD

Given South Sudan's challenges as a young country with a long history of conflicts that are still raging, sport will likely not be a significant priority for its government leaders and other stakeholders in the coming years. Yet, the role that sport can play in forging an identity that can unite disparate groups is also on people's minds. It is apparent on days such as in August, 2015, when the IOC announced South Sudan would be joining the Olympic family. It is apparent on days such as in April, 2016, at the Wrestling for Peace competition, when officials, athletes, and citizens express relief through sport from the violence that has marked their region for decades. Sport is not the sole answer for South Sudan any more than it is the answer for established countries that use sport in the role of diplomacy or development. The country still seems to be grappling with the assertion that "meaningful sports-based projects work best when sport is part of a greater joined-up picture or whole.

Sport and physical activity can play vital roles as agents of progress" (Jarvie, 2013). There is still no clearly stated intention for what the country's sport leaders will do to leverage sport. How will it maximize its strengths and find solutions for mitigating its weaknesses to find success on the playing field, and ensure that sport in South Sudan itself will be favorably experienced, and also lead to positive brand associations in Sudan, in Africa, and around the world?

It seems safe to say that when the history of South Sudan is written, how the country dealt with its youth will be one important factor. Another is understanding that diplomacy is just as much about forging an identity and expressing that identity (i.e., nation-branding) abroad; it doesn't have to be the traditional public diplomacy of winning hearts and minds. Judging from his quote below and other public comments since 2012, Miading Miaker already seems to understand the difference. When it comes to sport diplomacy for a troubled, fledgling nation, that contemporary view that sounds simple and not very significant can actually reap big rewards:

> A country like South Sudan, seeing me out there and the country just emerged and there's no sport, no facilities and everything just needs to be built, I think it's very important for South Sudan to have me there. Even though I wouldn't be the gold medalist or something like that, at least I would give them motivation a little bit. If I perform well at international competition, I think that would lift their spirits. (Gambaccini, 2013)

DISCUSSION QUESTIONS

1. Why is marathoner Guor Miading Miaker (formerly Guor Marial) a vibrant living symbol for the young country of South Sudan?

2. What are the distinctions between public diplomacy and nation branding? Which do you think is a more effective strategy for leaders of the young country of South Sudan?

3. What are South Sudan's strengths and weaknesses in attempting to develop a robust sporting infrastructure?

4. Despite its significant obstacles, are there advantages to being a new country such as South Sudan in forging an identity through sport that established nations don't enjoy?

5. What are some ways that South Sudan might take a traditional sport such as wrestling and use it to shape public opinion abroad more effectively than internationally accepted sports such as basketball, soccer, and athletics?

6. Do you interpret sport diplomacy differently in South Sudan's case than you did with other countries? How? And why?

REFERENCES

Annan, K., & Mousavizadeh, N. (2012). *Interventions: A life in war and peace*. London, UK: Allen and Lane.

Boboya, J. (2015). Assessing the context of youth civic engagement and leadership in South Sudan. *ResearchGate*. June. Retrieved from https://www.researchgate.net/profile/Boboya_James/publication/277912781_Assessing_the_Context_of_Youth_Civic_Engagement_and_Leadership_In_South_Sudan/links/55769c0408ae75363751b056.pdf

Coalter, F. (2010). The politics of sport-for-development: Limited focus programmes and broad gauge problems? *International Review for the Sociology of Sport, 45*, 295-314.

Collins, C. (2015). Luol Deng: South Sudan court among 'most memorable' accomplishments. *The Sporting News*, 9 Aug. Retrieved from http://www.sportingnews.com/nba-news/4652111-luol-deng-manute-bol-court-south-sudan-picture-instagram

Deng, F. M. (2001). Sudan—Civil war and genocide: Disappearing Christians of the Middle East. *Middle East Quarterly, 8*, 13-21. Retrieved from http://www.meforum.org/22/sudan-civil-war-and-genocide

De Souza, C. (2016). Fighting for peace in South Sudan. *Peace and Sport Watch*. (21 April). Retrieved from http://watch.peace-sport.org/fighting-for-peace-in-south-sudan/

Dewaal, A. (2012, July 2). Sudan and South Sudan's sporting chance. *World Peace Foundation*. Retrieved from http://sites.tufts.edu/reinventingpeace/2012/07/24/sudan-and-south-sudans-sporting-chance/

Dichter, H., & Johns, A. L., Eds. (2014). *Diplomatic games: Sport, statecraft, and international relations since 1945*. Lexington, Ky.: University Press of Kentucky.

Doherty, B. (2016). South Sudan Olympics chief says advertising deal swayed Rio team selection. *The Guardian*. 29 July. Retrieved from https://www.theguardian.com/sport/2016/jul/30/allegations-emerge-of-south-sudan-rio-team-selection-being-swayed-by-advertising-deal

Duff, B. (2016). Miami Heat star Deng to reach out to Nicola. *Windsor Star*. 4 May. Retrieved from http://windsorstar.com/sports/basketball/nba/nba-star-deng-to-reach-out-to-nicola

Edun, T. (2011). Sudan: Third civil war? The crisis in Abyei requires an immediate international response. *Institute for Policy Studies*. 1 June. Retrieved from http://www.ips-dc.org/sudan_third_civil_war/

Ensor, M. O. (2013). Youth culture, refugee (re)integration, and diasporic identities in South Sudan. *Postcolonial Text, 8*(3-4).

Fan, Y. (2006). Nation branding: What is being branded? *Journal of Vacation Marketing, 12*, 5-14.

Fortin, J. (2016, April 26). Riek Machar, South Sudan opposition leader, returns as part of peace deal. *New York Times*. Retrieved from http://www.nytimes.com/2016/04/27/world/africa/riek-machar-south-sudan-opposition-leader-returns-as-part-of-peace-deal.html?ribbon-ad-idx=4&rref=world/africa&module=Ribbon&version=context&region=Header&action=click&contentCollection=Africa&pgtype=article&_r=2

Gambaccini, P. (2013, March 11). New U.S. elite Guor Marial bears lessons of difficult upbringing. *Runner's World Newswire*. Retrieved from http://www.runnersworld.com/newswire/new-us-elite-guor-marial-bears-lessons-of-difficult-upbringing

Grohmann, K. (2015, August 2). South Sudan becomes Olympic Movement's 206th member. *Reuters*. Retrieved from https://uk.sports.yahoo.com/news/south-sudan-becomes-olympic-movements-206th-member-121212156--spt.html

Gudjonsson, H. (2005, March 2). Nation branding. *Place Branding. 1 issue#*, 283-98.

International Olympic Committee (2016, March 2). Team of refugee Olympic athletes created by the IOC (ROA). Retrieved from https://www.olympic.org/news/team-of-refugee-olympic-athletes-roa-created-by-the-ioc

Jarvie, G. (2013, January 29). War, peace and a new world paved with good intentions through sport. *E-International Relations*, Retrieved from http://www.e-ir.info/2013/01/29/war-peace-and-a-new-world-paved-with-good-intentions-through-sport/

Lomong, L. (2012). *Running for my life: One lost boy's journey from the killing fields of Sudan to the Olympic Games*. Nashville, TN: Thomas Nelson.

McConnell, T. (2011, July 11). South Sudan: Basketball star Luol Deng cheers independence. *GlobalPost*. Retrieved from http://www.globalpost.com/dispatch/news/regions/africa/110711/south-sudan-basketball-star-luol-deng-independence-juba-NBA

Murray, S. (2012). The two halves of sports-diplomacy. *Diplomacy & Statecraft. 23*, 576-92.

Omeje, K., & N. Minde. (2014). Stakeholder perspectives on priorities for postconflict state building and peace building in South Sudan. *Africa Peace & Conflict Journal, 7*, 14-28.

A policy strategy paper on youth employment creation and income generation in South Sudan. 2014. *Nyamilepdia*. 4 Dec. Retrieved from http://www.nyamile.com/2014/12/04/a-policy-strategy-paper-on-youth-employment-creation-and-income-generation-in-south-sudan/

Rice, X. (2011, July 8). Eight things you need to know about South Sudan. *The Guardian*. Retrieved from http://www.theguardian.com/world/2011/jul/08/south-sudan-eight-facts

Sharp, P. (1999). For diplomacy: Representation and the study of international relations. *International Studies Review, 1*, 33–57.

South Sudan rebel Riek Machar 'controls key state'. (2013, December 22). *BBC*. Retrieved from http://www.bbc.com/news/world-africa-25480178.

South Sudan to compete in Rio after becoming 206th Olympic nation. (2015, August 2). *The Guardian,* Retrieved from http://www.theguardian.com/world/2015/aug/02/south-sudan-compete-rio-206th-olympic-nation

Szondi, G. (2008). Public diplomacy and nation branding: Conceptual similarities and differences. *Discussion Papers in Diplomacy*. Netherlands Institute of International Relations 'Clingendael.' Retrieved from http://www.peacepalacelibrary.nl/ebooks/files/Clingendael_20081022_pap_in_dip_nation_branding.pdf

Wade, A. (2014, November 20). South Sudanese runner hoping to crowdfund his way to 2016 Olympics. *Runner's World Newswire*. Retrieved from http://www.runnersworld.com/newswire/south-sudanese-runner-hoping-to-crowdfund-his-way-to-2016-olympics

Ylönen, A (2012). Limits of 'peace through statebuilding' in southern Sudan: Challenges to state legitimacy, governance and economic development during the comprehensive peace agreement implementation, 2005-2011. *Journal of Conflictology, 3*(2), 28-40.

12

Sport as a Political Strategy in South-North Korean Relations

IK YOUNG CHANG

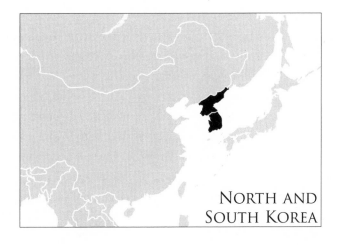

NORTH AND
SOUTH KOREA

INTRODUCTION

The vast majority of Koreans suffered under Japanese colonial rule for 36 years from 1910 to 1945. However, the United States-Soviet Union-led division of the nation at the 38th parallel in 1948 became a prelude to a sad history on the Korean peninsula. The division eventually led to the Korean War in 1950 and now Korea, along with Sudan and South Sudan (see "South Sudan's Quest for International Acceptance and Internal Identity through Sport") remain the only two divided nations in the world since both Germany and Yemen were reunified in 1990. For this reason, many countries around the world have watched in anticipation of a potential reunification and there have been continuous efforts to achieve this end from both the North and South Korean governments (Harrison, 2003).

Despite strong desire and effort for reunification both domestically and internationally, the 70-year-long history of inter-Korean division has created vast differences in political and economic systems that are difficult hurdles to surmount. However, Jonsson (2006) points out the importance of shared tradition and culture as an effective alternative to overcome political and economic heterogeneity in the context of the two Koreas.

A combination of a lengthy joint history from 668 to 1945, as well as the usage of a common language, ultimately contributes towards not only a sense of unity, but indeed a unified culture. This common language and these shared historical traditions create a symbolic mechanism for eventual re-integration of the currently heterogeneous ways of life pertaining on both sides of the border.

In the same vein, many scholars argue that sociocultural exchanges and cooperation help the divided nation to overcome the political distrust and animosity and to defuse the military tension and conflicts that have characterized inter-Korean relations since 1950 (Kim, Kim, Lee, & Yu, 2014; Jeon, 2006; Jung, 2013; Rhee, 1993). Indeed, while political and economic issues have been at the centre of the potential unification of the two Korean states, there has been no doubt that sociocultural exchanges and cooperation (including arts, religion, media, tourism, and sport) have played a catalytic role in solving a political impasse. In turn, sociocultural exchanges have contributed to development of inter-Korean relations and peace on the Korean peninsula.

Amongst the wide range of sociocultural exchanges and cooperation initiatives, sport has been frequently used as "a way to display shared cultural and national identity" (Lee, 2015, p. 2) because people believe that a sporting agenda may not raise political and ideological issues. Moreover, sport can be utilized as a pretext for opening formal diplomatic talks at a fraction of the cost when compared with other sociocultural exchanges. For instance, since the first official inter-Korean talks between South and North Korea were held in August 1971, there have been a total of 55 sociocultural dialogues. More specifically, 47 of those dialogues were related to sports exchanges and cooperation, therefore accounting for more than 85% of the total negotiations (Korean Ministry of Unification, 2015). Thus, sport has occupied a significant position within the context of politics and diplomatic relations. As a cultural site and practice, sport in contemporary society has been a part of both domestic and international politics (Allison, 1993; Hoberman, 1984; Houlihan, 2007; Jackson, 2013). Similarly, Jung (2013, p. 308) points out that "modern sport has been constructed by the demands of the state and capital, which in turn intensifies its role both as a method of political image manipulation domestically and as a tool of diplomacy externally."

However, sport is a double-edged sword in the context of wider political and diplomatic practice (Marks, 1998). On the one hand, sport can serve as a focus that assists in the initiation of conflict between countries. The most famous example of this phenomenon is that of the "Football War" between Honduras and El Salvador in 1969, which tragically resulted in the deaths of approximately 3,000 civilians and the creation of hundreds of thousands of refugees from both countries. On the other hand, there are numerous examples of the way in which sport has functioned to help to facilitate cooperation and build trust by bridging the differences between hostile countries. For instance, ping-pong diplomacy led to Richard Nixon's visit to China in 1972 when ideological confrontation between the Western and Eastern Blocs was at its height. Another example is that of "wrestling diplomacy" which helped to foster a completely new relationship between Iran and the USA following the Iran hostage crisis which lasted for 444 days between 1979-1981 (see "Wrestling with Diplomacy: The US and Iran").

The role of sport in the international context can be equally applied to the two Koreas' context. During the peak of the Cold War period of the 1960s to 1970s, sport was a mirror of the political conflict and ideological feud between South and North Korea. As a result, both nation-states strategically invested enormous capital into elite sport under the belief that winning more medals at a variety of international sporting events might reflect the superiority of one political system over the other.

In contrast to the role of sport as a symbol of the political and ideological conflict, sport has also been used as a means for recovering the social and cultural homogeneity of North and South Korea (Markel, 2008, 2009; Lee, 2010, 2015). The end of the Cold War in the 1980s contributed to the harmony of the Eastern and Western blocs and also affected the South-North relations. For instance, the South Korean government made efforts to restore relations with communist countries, including North Korea, and the 1990 Asian Games in Beijing gave both Koreas a great opportunity to improve relations with their counterpart. During the period of the 1990 Beijing Asian Games, South and North Korea agreed to hold unification football matches in Seoul and Pyongyang in October, 1990. The friendly matches provided a cornerstone for creating an amicable environment between the two Koreas and finally led to the formation of a unified Korean team for the World Table Tennis Championships in Chiba, Japan, in April, 1991 and for the FIFA World Youth Championships in Portugal in June, 1991.

However, a mood of reconciliation did not last long because of the political and military conflicts from both Koreas. In other words, the frozen political relations between the two Koreas deeply affected inter-Korean sports exchanges and cooperation. Therefore, the joy and grief of the sporting exchanges between the two Koreas has been reflective of changing governmental and political circumstances. To date, previous research has focused on the positive and apolitical role of sport and overly emphasized the instrumental value of sport in inter-Korean relations. However, there has been little research on how the political intentions and decisions have affected inter-Korean sport exchanges and cooperation. Therefore, this study focuses on how the two Koreas have used sport talks and exchanges as part of a wider political strategy to achieve their own aims at different times.

The remainder of this case study is divided into three sections to guide analysis. First is a brief historical context of the two Koreas. Second is a review of the variety of reunification policies in inter-Korean relations and an examination of the role of sport exchanges as a wider strategy to achieve the political goals pursued by the South and North Korean governments. Third, is a discussion regarding the contribution of political relations to sport exchanges in inter-Korean relations.

FROM ONE KOREA TO TWO:
UNDERSTANDING THE CONTEXTS

Korea has a long history, spanning thousands of years, having endured almost 1,000 instances of invasion by its powerful neighbors such as China, Japan, and Russia. Although there have been many changes in the names of the various dynasties throughout Korea's long history, such as Kochoson (ancient Chosun: B.C. 2,333-B.C. 108); Three Kingdoms (B.C. 50-668), including Koguryo, Paekche and Silla; Unified Silla (668-918); Koryo Dynasty (918-1392); and Choson Dynasty (1392-1910). Korea has maintained, ethnically and culturally, a relatively homogeneous state for over five millennia.

At the end of the nineteenth century, conflicts over Korea between China, Russia, and Japan led to the outbreak of the 1894-1895 Sino-Japanese War and the 1904-1905 Russo-Japanese War, both of which ended with Japan's victory and in turn, helped reinforce Japan's political influence in the Peninsula. As a result, Japan declared Korea as a protectorate in 1905, and five years later as a colony under the annexation treaty. Japan ruled Korea until its surrender to the Allied forces on August 15, 1945 (Kim, 1962).

Soon after World War II, the United States and the Soviet Union agreed to a temporary division of the Korean Peninsula based on the Thirty-eighth Parallel. However, the emerging Cold War dashed hopes for a unified Korea and each division established their own state: the Republic of Korea (South Korea) and the Democratic People's Republic of Korea (North Korea) in August and September 1948, respectively. The division eventually led to the Korean War (1950-1953), resulting in the deaths of millions of soldiers and civilians together with massive destruction of social and physical infrastructure. A demilitarized zone (DMZ) across the Korean Peninsula was established in July 1953.

Since 1953, the homogenous culture that had endured for 5,000 years has been radically changed by the vastly different political and economic systems of the two Koreas. North Korea has been heavily affected by the communist regime. At the same time, however, North Korea developed an official ideology, self-reliance (*juche*), based on political independence, economic self-sustenance, and self-reliance in defence, strengthening the role of the Great Leader and justifying the hereditary succession from Kim Il-sung to Kim Jong-il to Kim Jong-un (Armstrong, 2005; Lim, 2012). This rigid state-controlled system has helped the dictators to consolidate their political and military power, but it has also led to a severe economic crisis since 1990. Economic deprivation has been accelerated by repeated natural disasters that have caused chronic food shortages and lead North Korea to make requests for humanitarian assistance from international organizations, including South Korea.

South Korea, on the other hand, has maintained strong political, economic, and military relationships with the United States. The South Korean government has achieved remarkable economic achievements since the 1960s. In addition, South Korea successfully hosted the 1988 Seoul Olympics, which not only helped the country showcase their rise from a poor state ruined by the Korean War to a modern, industrial and democratic state, but also contributed to restoring its relations with other countries—in particular, communist countries such as the Soviet Union and China. Although South Korea has faced the global economic crisis and ideological issues both domestically and globally, the nation has managed to achieve significant political and economic development within the context of the compressed modernity (Chang, 1999).

Despite the vastly different contexts of the two Koreas since the 1950s (which affects the balance and power in inter-Korean relations), the dynamic relationship between South and North Korea has made it possible to produce a variety of reunification policies, including sporting exchanges and cooperation. Therefore, the next section reviews the variety of reunification policies in inter-Korean relations and explores how sporting exchanges play a role as a vehicle for facilitating cooperation and reconciliation or creating tensions and conflicts between two Koreas.

INTER-KOREAN RELATIONS: SPORT AS A POLITICAL STRATEGY

Since the establishment of separate governments in South and North Korea in 1948, inter-Korean relations have fluctuated. Scholars have pointed out that there are four main factors that have affected inter-Korean relations: (a) the political situation in the two Koreas, (b) the end of the Cold War, (c) the discrepancy in economic development between the two Koreas, and (d) North Korea's nuclear weapon issue (Heo & Roehrig, 2014; Jung, 2013).

Drawing upon these four factors, Heo and Roehrig (2014) assert that inter-Korean relations can be divided into four different periods: (a) antagonistic period (1953 to 1987), when ideological confrontation was at its height and, as a result, there were frequent military clashes between the South and North Korea; (b) coexistence period (1988 to 1997), when the Cold War ended and the two Koreas joined the UN; (c) engagement policy period (1998 to 2007), when inter-Korean relations were improved by the "Sunshine" policy, which "can be seen as a proactive policy to induce incremental and voluntary changes in North Korea for peace, opening and reform through the patient pursuit of reconciliation, exchanges and cooperation" (Moon, 2002, p. 27); and (d) conditional engagement policy period (2008 to present) when the presidents from the conservative party regarded the Sunshine policy as a failure and tensions in the Korean peninsula were escalated by North Korea military provocations, such as the sinking of a South Korean warship and the shelling of Yeongyeong Island.

The paper will now review the political strategies that have been utilized to hold a dominant position in inter-Korean relations from the South and North states and explore how sport has been used as part of wider political strategies.

ANTAGONISTIC PERIOD (1953-1987)

Based on a degree of antagonistic confrontation, the antagonistic period, beginning from the Korean War armistice of 1953 until the authoritarian regime of the Fifth Republic under President Chun Doo-Hwan in 1987, can be classified into two phases: (a) antagonistic confrontation from 1953 to 1971, when the Cold War reached its height and, as a result, there were a number of military clashes between the two Koreas; and (b) antagonistic deadlock from 1971 to 1987, when the two governments opened official dialogues that focused primarily on achieving the political pretext and successful propaganda.

ANTAGONISTIC CONFRONTATION PHASE (1953-1971)

For almost two decades after an armistice agreement in 1953, both the two Koreas had been engaged in antagonistic confrontation, not only through military clashes but also in political, economic, and diplomatic issues. For instance, there have been 193 inter-Korean military clashes recorded in the media between 1955 and 2010. Among them, 62 incidents took place during this antagonistic confrontation period, accounting for almost a third of military clashes. In the political and diplomatic realm, neither of the two states recognized their rival's existence nor established diplomatic relations with foreign countries that recognized their opponent. In other words, inter-Korean relations were completely influenced by the tension and conflict between the Cold War Blocs, as each Korea was tightly anchored to the United States and Soviet Union respectively.

Until the end of the 1960s, high-risk confrontation on the Korean peninsula continued to rise because both South and North Korea would not relinquish military force as a tool to solve the issue of reunification. As a result, contact between South and North Korea had been virtually nonexistent.

Despite severe confrontation, the two Koreas both recognized sport as a means to showcase their political, economic, and cultural superiority on the international stage. While the National Olympic Committee in South Korea (SKOC) was recognized by the International Olympic Committee (IOC) before the Korean War, North Korea did not even have an opportunity to promote their elite athletic performers on the grounds that there could not be more than one recognized NOC in any one country (Hill, 1996).

In 1957, therefore, the communist state unofficially proposed to form a unified team for the 1960 Rome Olympics to their counterpart and, at the same time, the Eastern bloc put pressure on the IOC to give provisional recognition for the North under the premise that the two Koreas should form a unified team for the 1960 Rome Olympics. North Korea's proposal on forming a unified team suddenly disappeared when North Korea achieved their goal and obtained IOC membership. However, as the IOC gave the North Korean National Olympic Committee (NKOC) a conditional membership, which limited "the boundary of North Korea's Olympic Committee to inside its own territory" (Jung, 2013, p. 311), North Korea made a proposal for holding South-North sport talks in order to obtain full and separate recognition for international events again. In January, 1963, the two Koreas held the first talks in Lausanne, Switzerland, under the arbitration of the IOC with the support of the Cold War Blocs and follow-up meetings were held in Hong Kong in May and July, 1973, without formal IOC participation. Although it was unofficial and no real progress was made during these talks, it should be noted that the historic first meeting after the division laid the foundation for inter-Korean relations, and sport occupied a prominent place in the process.

ANTAGONISTIC DEADLOCK PERIOD (1971-1987)

The global situation changed drastically in the early 1970s when Richard Nixon became the first United States President to visit China (North Korea's closest ally), after the invitation of U.S. table tennis players in what became known as ping-pong diplomacy (see "Introduction: A Review of How Sports Can Be Used to Improve International Relationships" and "The U.S. Government's Role in Sport Diplomacy"). In addition to dramatic changes in the external environment, the South and North Korean governments modified their reunification policy. The South Korean government focused on economic growth because the authoritarian government in the South believed that economic development could be a tool to prevent another North Korea attack. North Korea proposed a new approach on Korean reunification by forming a federation between South and North Korea-"one country, two political systems, each retaining its economic system-for both Koreas" (Heo & Roehrig, 2014, p.31). In other words, South and North Korea realized that unification by force was no longer possible.

Such changes, both domestically and globally, led to face-to-face inter-Korean dialogue. The first official South and North dialogue began with a humanitarian issue in August, 1971, when the South Korean Red Cross proposed the reunion of separated families to the North Korean Red Cross. Following the humanitarian talks, the two governments constructed a secret channel for high-level contacts and the two sides finally agreed via the joint communiqué of July 4, 1972, which included three principles for reunification between South and North Korea (Ministry of Unification, 2015):

(1) Reunification will take place without reliance on or intervention by foreign nations; it will be achieved by a peaceful means.

(2) The two sides shall take measures to stop propaganda broadcasting against the other side, stop military aggression and prevent any military clashes.

(3) The two sides shall institute various exchanges in the economic, social and cultural areas; cooperate in holding inter-Korean Red Cross talks; open a Seoul-Pyongyang hotline; and set up a South-North mediation committee.

As a result of the communiqué, the two Koreas established the South-North Coordinating Committee (NSCC) and a direct telephone hotline at Panmunjeom, which is located in the middle of the DMZ, for a meeting between the South and North.

However, a mood of reconciliation between the two Koreas did not last long because rulers of the two Koreas wanted to take absolute power through the Yushin constitution passed in October, 1972, in the South and the Kim Il-Sung idolization campaign in the early 1970s in the North. This deadlock situation interrupted building a cooperative system through dialogues and continued until 1979 when South Korean President Park Chung-hee was assassinated. Although there had been 121 political, humanitarian, and sociocultural meetings, talks, and negotiations, including sport dialogues, between the South and North

Korea from 1971 to 1979, their efforts proved fruitless. Indeed, the strategy used by the two Koreas at that time was always to object to each other's proposals, as they believed that having a constructive dialogue for their mutual interest would not help retain their regime.

During this period, South and North Korea exchanged a variety of ideas and perspectives on sport. In 1972 the presidents of the SKOC and NKOC issued a joint statement about forming a unified team for the 1972 Munich Olympics and the president of the South Korean Football Association invited officials from the North Korean Football Association to cooperate in a good-will match in 1976. In 1978 when the South Koreans hosted the first international sporting event, the 42nd ISSF World Shooting Championship, the government officially announced that they would invite North Korea to Seoul. Less than a year later, North Korea proposed forming a unified team for the 35th World Table Tennis Championship and the 1980 Moscow Olympics.

In spite of all these efforts to hold various inter-Korean sports exchanges, sport-based diplomatic initiatives did not make a significant positive contribution to the development of inter-Korean relations. Sport remained as a tool of political propaganda for proving the superiority of their respective systems. Indeed, each Korea always made unilateral proposals with no respect or regard for the other.

After October 26, 1979, following the assassination of President Park Chung-hee, who governed the country for 18 years, General Chun Doo-whan seized power through the 12·12 coup in 1979. The military leader tried to justify the new administration by enhancing economic growth and promoting the 3S "Sex, Sports and Screen" policy, taking public interest away from domestic politics. Externally the authoritarian regime also tried to build a close relationship with the United States, emphasizing the importance of national security, while proposing summit talks to North Korean leader, Kim Il-sung who had already achieved absolute power. However, North Korea's response was an attempted bombing attack in Rangoon, Burma (Myanmar), in 1983 to assassinate President Chun, which failed but killed 17 South Korean officials.

Despite North Korea's hostile reaction, the South Korea government continuously proposed humanitarian aid for a series of natural disasters in North Korea in the mid-1980s. Unlike their previous response, surprisingly, North Korea accepted the offer and both Koreas reopened the Red Cross talks on a reunion of separated families in 1984. As a result of the talks, separated family members, 35 from South Korea and 30 from North Korea, visited Seoul and Pyongyang respectively in September 1985. However, inter-Korean relations did not develop further due to North Korea's absurd requests, such as suspension of the joint military training between the US and South Korea and the abolition of National Security Law. Moreover, a bomb blast at Gimpo International Airport in Seoul, which killed five and wounded over 30 others in September 1986, and the explosion of Korean Air flight 858 in November 1987, which killed 115 passengers and crew members (both of which were committed by North Korea), made inter-Korean relations worse.

According to Lee (2002), sport in the 1980s played a significant role in creating political conflicts between the South and North. Indeed, the IOC's 1981 decision to award the rights to host the 1988 Olympic Games to Seoul was regarded as a serious threat to North Korea "as [North Korea] perceived it as proof of system supremacy of the South" (Jung, 2013: 313). Under this circumstance, North Korea adopted two different approaches in sports exchanges with South Korea. One was to sabotage the successful hosting of international sporting events such as the 1986 Asian Games and 1988 Olympics in Seoul by creating an atmosphere of terror and boycotting with other communist countries. The main aim of a series of North Korean bombings in Burma, Seoul, and KAL 858 flight was to hinder the successful delivery of the international sporting events held in Seoul, South Korea. In addition, North Korea was systematically involved in the boycott of both sporting events, persuading their communist allies to stay home. However, North Korea's violent and irrational behaviour faced condemnation from neighbouring countries and left an indelible stain on their reputation.

On the other hand, North Korea continuously called for sport talks in an effort to negotiate co-hosting the Games with South Korea. North Korea had already recognized that its allies (including the Soviet Union and China) did not support the boycott of the Seoul Olympic Games. By having negotiations with South Korea and advocating co-hosting the Games, North Korea was attempting to ingratiate itself with the people of South Korea and the international community. However, the North demanded too much of the IOC and the South Korean government. For example, North Korea proposed that the Games should be labelled as Chosun or Pyongyang-Seoul Olympics, the number of Olympic events should be equally hosted in both states, and the broadcast revenue should be equally distributed to the two Koreas. North Korea's proposals were rejected by both the IOC and South Korea, but as part of its efforts to have a successful Olympic Games, the IOC proposed that five Olympic events, such as archery, table tennis, women's volleyball, a preliminary round of the soccer competition, and the men's individual cycling road race, could be hosted in the North (Ha, 1998). In June 1986 when the South and North held their third meeting, both states accepted the IOC proposal, but one year later North Korea finally rejected it because free travel of athletes and the general public during the Olympic period between the North and South through the Demilitarized Zone (DMZ) might threaten North Korea's political system.

Throughout the antagonistic period, sport was another political battlefield. Indeed, sport talks and exchanges between the North and South remained at the level of political propaganda for South and North Korea. For example, sport talks related to forming a unified team for the Olympic Games and co-hosting international sporting events, such as the 1986 Asian Games and 1988 Olympic Games held in Seoul, played a substantive role in political negotiation between the two Koreas, offering a unique space where they could show off the supremacy of their respective political, ideological, and diplomatic systems. Therefore, the history of inter-Korean relations in sport from 1953 to 1987 had worked politically at different times despite the claim that sport was an apolitical or depoliticized site within society.

COEXISTENCE PERIOD (1988-1997)

Inter-Korean relations unexpectedly changed in the late 1980s for two main reasons: (1) the end of the Cold War and (2) the increased gap in economic growth between the two Koreas. The new world order after the Cold War paved a way for harmony between the Eastern and Western blocs and affected the Korean peninsula, the world's last frontier of the Cold War. In order to quickly and efficiently deal with the situation, Roh Tae-woo, the political successor of the previous authoritarian leader in South Korea, Chun Doo-whan, tried to build new and close ties with former communist countries, including the Soviet Union and China by proposing economic aid and exchanges, known as Nord Politik (Northern Policy). The Northern Policy helped to establish diplomatic relations with the Soviet Union and China in 1990 and 1992 respectively.

South Korea achieved rapid economic growth from the 1960s through the early 1990s, while North Korea's economy was stuck at the same level as in the 1970s. South Korea's economic development contributed to building its strong national security. Therefore, South Korea's economic and military superiority helped to foster the belief in South Koreans that war is unlikely to happen on the Korea peninsula.

With such radical changes occurring, the South Korean government announced the Declaration for National Self-Esteem, Unification, and Prosperity in July, 1988. This declaration aimed at not only easing the tension and conflict, but also at building a partnership with North Korea, and played an important role in improving inter-Korean relations. Indeed, it led to the first prime ministerial talks in September 1990 and South and North Korea became members of the UN separately in September 1991, officially recognizing each other's political system. In February 1992, the two Koreas reached the Joint Declaration on the Denuclearization, which contributed to peace on the Korean peninsula (Seth, 2010), and the Roh government cancelled a combined South-U.S. military exercise, the "Team Spirit," in hopes North Korea would abandon its nuclear program and accept the International Atomic Energy Agency's (IAEA) inspections.

Kim Young-sam, the president of the first civilian government in South Korea, inherited the Roh government's peaceful coexistence policy toward North Korea. However, the issue of North Korea's withdrawal from the Nuclear Non-Proliferation Treaty (NTP) hindered the government's efforts to improve inter-Korean relations. To solve this problem, the U.S. administration decided to intervene and sent the former U.S. president Jimmy Carter as a presidential envoy to North Korea. He had a meeting with Kim Il-sung, and they agreed that North Korea would stop its nuclear program and allow IAEA special inspections. After Carter's visit, North Korea proposed high-level talks to the US, and in October 1994 they signed the agreed framework.

South Korea and North Korea also reached an agreement to the summit meeting, but it was cancelled due to Kim Il-sung's sudden death in July 1994. His death aggravated inter-Korean relations as the Kim administration not only refused to offer condolences, but also prohibited private condolences to Kim Il-sung's death. To lessen this tension, the South

Korean government provided food aid to North Korea, asking for the talks. It was not only South Korea's first direct economic aid to the North since the division, but the first attempt to use economic assistance as a diplomatic means to improve inter-Korean relations (Bae & Myong, 2011).

The successful hosting of the 1988 Seoul Olympic Games also helped to reopen the lines of communication between the two Koreas. In December, the president of the NKOC first proposed sport talks on a unified team for the 11th Beijing Asian Games. Between March 1989 to February 1990, both Koreas had nine regular sessions and six working-level talks, but did not reach a final agreement because of "different opinions on the formality of the agreement and assurance of performance on the agreed agenda" (Jung, 2013, p. 316).

Although the two Koreas failed to form an inter-Korean team for international mega-sporting events, they learned how to negotiate with each other. During the Beijing Asian Games, the South and North Korean Ministers of Sport met and agreed to having a South-North unification football goodwill games with the first games held in Pyongyang from 9 to 13 October, 1990 and then in Seoul from 21 to 25 October, 1990 (Chung, 1998). At the end of the games, both states announced they would continue open dialogue about forming a unified team.

In November, 1991 they met to discuss the issue of participating in the international sporting events as one team and, finally, ping-pong diplomacy version 2.0 arrived in Korea. This agreement led to the formation of a unified table tennis team for the first time after the division for the 41st World Table Tennis Championships held in Chiba, Japan, in April, 1991. Moreover, they also sent a unified team for the 6th World Junior Soccer Championships held in Portugal in June 1991. Both agreements, which formed a unified team under the "Team Korea," were historic events for Korean and for the world.

The new world order after the Cold War ended, and South Korea's dramatic economic development made North Korea feel that the North's political ideological system had fallen behind the South's both domestically and internationally. For North Korea, therefore, there was no other option but to artificially have the inter-Korean sport exchange, which seemed a far less difficult political issue to manage when compared to the other political and economic crises. In other words, trying to improve inter-Korean relations through sport exchanges and talks gave North Korea opportunities to overcome the international isolation and economic difficulties and to present a new image around the globe. Consequently, sport at that time was used as a common space where North Korea could escape from political and economic difficulties, and South Korea could lead inter-Korean dialogue based on the superior position of their economic system.

ENGAGEMENT POLICY PERIOD (1998-2007)

In February, 1998, when a long-time democratic activist in South Korea, Kim Dae-jung, was elected the president of South Korea, inter-Korean relations were vastly improved by the Sunshine policy, which promoted greater engagement with North Korea (Moon, 2002).

This policy had three "P principles"—peaceful coexistence, peaceful exchange, and peaceful unification"—and three rules: "(1) no tolerance for any type of armed provocation, (2) no intention to harm or absorb North Korea and (3) to push reconciliation and cooperation between the two Koreas" (Heo & Roehrig, 2014, pp.37-38). The principles and rules contributed to building trust between the North and South through reconciliation and cooperation. This was the first policy that separated economics from politics.

In addition, the Sunshine policy eventually led to the first summit meeting between the leaders of the two Koreas in Pyongyang, the capital of North Korea, from 13-15 June 2000. On the last day of the summit meeting, Kim Dae-jung and Kim Jong-il signed a joint declaration, known as the 6.15 declaration, which included (a) solving reunification issues independently through the joint efforts of the Korean people; (b) finding a common element in the South's concept of a confederation and the North's formula for a loose form of federation; (c) promptly resolving humanitarian issues such as separated family members and unswerving communists serving prison sentences in the South; (d) building mutual trust by promoting balanced economic development through cooperation and by stimulating cooperation and exchanges in other fields such as culture, health, environment, and sports; and (e) holding high-level talks in the near future to implement the above agreements (BBC, 2000). Based on the declaration, both Koreas held a minister-level meeting and agreed to ease military conflict and to remove the risk of war.

The principle of separation of political matters from economic matters allowed South Korea to send 200,000 tons of fertilizer to North Korea in April 2002 and to build a joint industrial complex that was deemed vital for North Korean's economy in Kaesong, North Korea, in June 2003. The summit meeting and follow-up actions played an important role in changing South Koreans' perception of North Korea. As time went by, however, this policy faced public criticism because North Korea was only interested in receiving economic aid from South Korea rather than in building mutual confidence in other fields, especially in politics and the military.

Despite North Korea's ongoing nuclear weapon threat and naval clashes in the Yellow Sea between South and North Korea, Kim Dae-jung's successor, Roh Moo-hyun, maintained the framework of the previous government's policy toward North Korea under a different name, the Peace and Prosperity policy (Bae & Myong, 2011). This policy included four main rules: (a) the two Koreas resolve all controversial issues through dialogue; (b) build mutual confidence and uphold reciprocity; (c) agree to cooperate internationally in inter-Korean relations as the main actors; and (d) improve transparency and accountability in South-North relations (Funabashi, 2007). Like the previous government, the Roh administration also proclaimed that the policy toward North Korea would separate humanitarian assistance from political issues. As a result, the government provided $385 million worth of humanitarian aid to the North, including food and fertilizer.

In 2007 there was the second summit meeting between the South and North that confirmed the implementation of the 6.15 joint declaration. However, North Korea's first nuclear test and a long-range missile test in 2006 aggravated inter-Korean relations and the engagement policy of ten years faced a great deal of criticism from the public. It should be noted that the Roh government's Peace and Prosperity policy was different from Kim Dae-jung's Sunshine policy because there already existed a negative circumstance created by the nuclear crisis. Therefore, the government took two different tracks toward the North in order to implement the Peace and Prosperity policy. While the Ministry of Unification worked to improve inter-Korean cooperation through economic and cultural exchanges, the Ministry of Foreign Affairs and Trade put political pressure on the North to stop their nuclear program (Snyder, 2005).

During both the Roh Tae-woo and Kim Young-sam governments, inter-Korean sport exchanges and cooperation had been more improved when compared to the authoritarian administrations in the past. As mentioned before, however, Kim Dae-jung and Roh Moo-hyun governments would not link cooperation and exchanges in other fields to political issues and in turn, this made it possible for both Koreas to have more active cooperation with each other in the field of sport. It should be noted that private enterprise played an important role in sport exchanges during the period. Chung Ju-yung, who was the founder of Hyundai and one of the biggest advocates for inter-Korean economy projects, built a sports complex in Pyongyang in 1999. His global corporation, Hyundai, held South-North Basketball Goodwill Games to celebrate starting construction of the building. Samsung also organized the Unification Table Tennis Goodwill Games at the Pyongyang gymnasium in July, 2000.

After the first summit meeting between the South and North in June 2000, the most astonishing result in South-North sport exchanges was a joint parade at the opening ceremony of the 2000 Sydney Olympic Games. Athletes and officials from the South and North Korea marched together hand in hand under the flag of the Korean peninsula for the first time since the division of Korea, but both Koreas competed separately in actual sporting events.

In 2002 another historical event occurred in inter-Korean sport exchanges. North Korea sent 318 athletes, 22 officials, and 355 cheerleaders to the 14th Asian Games held in South Korea. Prior to this event, North Korea had boycotted any international sporting events taking place in South Korea because the North regime had continuously denied South Korea's political legitimacy. In the same year, South and North Taekwondo demonstration teams visited Seoul and Pyongyang respectively and the two Koreas also held a conference to overcome the differences in terminologies, rules, and styles between the International Taekwondo Federation (ITF) and World Taekwondo Federation (WTF). One year later, Daegu Universiad Organizing Committee officially invited North Korea. In return, the North sent it's largest-ever team in North Korea's Universiad history to Daegu, South Korea. At the Athens Olympics in 2004, South and North Korea entered the main stadium together at the opening and closing ceremonies.

A series of sport exchanges within the private and public sector facilitated sociocultural cooperation between both Koreas and contributed to developing a mood of reconciliation on the Korean peninsula during the peak years of North Korea's nuclear weapon crisis. During the engagement period, it was recognized that sporting exchanges between South Korea and North Korea were a big contributor to the improvement of inter-Korean relations, in part due to relatively minor political interference. However, this was not a real mutual benefit resulting from a cooperation of the two Koreas, but rather an outcome of unilateral concessions made by South Korea, which made it possible for both Koreas to talk within the context of reconciliation. Indeed, the Kim Dae-jung and Roh Moo-hyun governments in South Korea tried to open the door to North Korea through their policies of unconditional provision toward North Korea such as the Sunshine policy and the Peace and Prosperity policy. The assumption was that the North regime just needed some time "to overcome international isolation and economic difficulties by selectively accepting the limited contacts and preferred exchanges" (Jung, 2013,p. 321). Thus, it is argued that sport was not at the forefront in inter-Korean exchanges, but rather, after political decisions were made, it was used strategically as a useful tool for fulfilling policy goals pursued by the two Korean governments.

CONDITIONAL ENGAGEMENT POLICY PERIOD (2008-PRESENT)

After the inauguration of the Lee Myung-bak government in South Korea, despite the huge improvement of inter-Korean relations under the leadership of Kim and Roh (1998-2008), the engagement policy was regarded as a failure because of South Korea's unilateral concessions and North Korea's unchanged attitude. Indeed, North Korea's lack of reciprocity and stance in relation to the nuclear issue had been at the centre of the controversy regarding the engagement policy. Therefore, the Lee government announced a revised engagement policy, the so-called "No Nuclear, Opening, 3,000 Plan," demanding denuclearization and emphasizing reciprocity as an essential precondition for further inter-Korean cooperation and exchanges.

In reality, South Korea stopped sending fertilizer in 2008 and reduced the economic assistance to its counterpart. A series of economic sanctions would send a strong message to the North to return to dialogue to discuss denuclearization and economic and cultural cooperation between the two Koreas. Unlike the South's hope, however, South-North relations were further aggravated. In July, 2008, a North Korean soldier shot and killed a South Korean visitor to the Mount Kumgang resort. The South Korean government immediately banned all tourists from visiting North Korea.

Moreover, tensions and conflicts on the Korean peninsula were further raised by North Korea military provocations such as the second nuclear test in May, 2009, the sinking of a South Korean warship in March, 2010, and the shelling of Yeongyeong Island in November 2010. In response to North Korea's military provocations, the Lee government halted all trade and aid to the North including humanitarian assistance. As a result, the relationship between the North and South descended to the worst point since the end of the Cold War as the Lee government held firm to the basic principles of its North Korea policy.

Park Geun-hye, Lee's political successor, kept in step with Lee's policy toward North Korea. In particular, her policy known as "the Korean Peninsula Trust Process" was very similar, in principle, to the economic and humanitarian aid after denuclearization. However,

Park's policy was more flexible when approaching denuclearization. She did not demand denuclearization as a precondition for economic aid, but rather tried to open a new era with the North through economic cooperation.

The Park government revised its North Korean policy as a response to the third nuclear test. This revised policy can simply be understood by the old saying, "An eye for an eye, a tooth for a tooth." For example, after North Korea conducted its third nuclear test, the South Korean government imposed stronger sanctions on North Korea by pulling all South Korean workers out of the Kaesong Industrial Complex. More recently, when North Korea fired a rocket and shells across the border into Yeoncheon County, which is close to the DMZ, the South military immediately responded by firing artillery shells in August 2015.

The changes to the political climate on the Korean peninsula, such as a new policy toward North Korea and its frequent provocations, significantly affected inter-Korean sport exchanges. In particular, during the Lee government (2008-2012), there were no sport exchanges between the South and North. Even an agreement on a unified team for the 2008 Beijing Olympic Games between the Roh Moo-hyun government and Kim Jong-il regime was cancelled.

However, when the Park administration eased the policy toward North Korea, compared to the previous Lee government, North Korea expressed its intention to send its athletes and cheerleaders to the 2014 Incheon Asian Games. The South Korean government accepted, expecting that this sporting initiative might improve the strained relationship with the North. In turn, North Korea requested financial assistance for athletes and cheerleaders during the Games, but South Korea refused their request based on "international standards under which countries cover the costs of their own traveling athletes" (The Guardian, 2014). After this meeting, even though North Korea finally agreed to participate in the Games, its cheerleaders could not travel alongside athletes.

In contrast to the 2002 Pusan Asian Games, the organizing committee and South Korean government treated the team from the North equally with the other 45 countries participating in the Games. There were no surprising events, such as a joint march at the opening ceremony or a display of the North Korean flag on the street (Lee, 2015). Unlike previous positive reactions to North Korean participation, there was no special treatment in the 2014 Inchon Asian Games, which may reflect strained South-North Korean relations.

On the final day of the Games, three high-level North Korean politicians, including the regime's second most powerful man, made a surprise visit to attend the closing ceremony. Their arrival raised hopes for a breakthrough in the frozen inter-Korean relations and helped resume high-level talks between the two Koreas. In this sense, sports can be viewed as a useful catalyst to reopen a blocked conversation channel between the South and North before other, higher order political decisions. However, this notion does not take into account the political benefits that North Korea can obtain when sending its top officials to the sporting event. At that time, North Korea was internationally isolated by UN sanctions for its nuclear test and also faced economic difficulties (BBC, 2000). To escape from this predicament, North Korea needed to change the situation, and sending high-ranking

A North Korean gymnast on the podium in the 2014 Incheon Asian Games, South Korea.

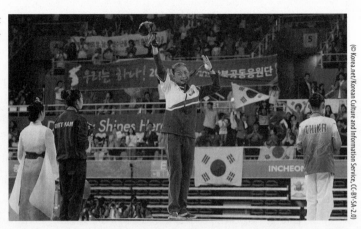

officials to the closing ceremony of the Asian Games held in South Korea was a good political strategy because, generally, sporting events have been regarded as apolitical from the public's viewpoint.

CONCLUSION

The political intentions and decisions between the South and North Korea have affected its sport exchanges and cooperation. More specifically, there has been a range of political strategies used in inter-Korean relations in an attempt by both countries to assert their dominance and superiority through sport. Thus, sport has been used as a part of wider governmental political strategies in inter-Korean relations.

It is clear that inter-Korean sport exchanges have reflected wider political strategies. Indeed, the fluctuating political situations between the two Koreas tend to be mirrored through the sport exchanges. In that sense, it could be argued that inter-Korean sport exchanges operate as a barometer of political decision-making at that particular time.

In addition, even though there has been research on the meaningful role of sport in politics and diplomacy, we must not overestimate the effect of sport on facilitating reconciliation and cooperation or creating conflict and tension. Sport did not bring about the South-North Korean exchanges through bottom-up processes (e.g., community and civil sector engagement between the two countries), but rather only after top-down governmental political decisions by one or both of the states were made. Indeed, sport was instrumentally used as a tool for fulfilling the political goals pursued by the South and North Korean governments. Therefore, in contrast to previous arguments that adopted a functional approach to sports' role in inter-Korean relations, it should be noted that sport exchanges have not been featured as the starting point to induce cooperation and reconciliation on the Korean peninsula. Rather, sport has been used as a tool for achieving the political strategies set by both states. Indeed, it is clear that sport has occupied a significant position within South-North Korean relations; however, it is important to recognize that the sporting exchanges were politically motivated and intentional in order to achieve a predetermined political strategy.

DISCUSSION QUESTIONS

1. Amongst the wide range of sociocultural exchanges why do people believe that sport can play such an important role in the development of inter-Korean relations?

2. Explain two contradictory roles of sport in the context of wider political and diplomatic relations.

3. What is the core role of sport in inter-Korean relations during the peak period of the Cold War?

4. Explain the effect of hosting the 1988 Seoul Olympic Games on South-North Korean relations.

5. How did the end of the Cold War contribute to both reviving South-North relations and developing inter-Korean sports exchanges?

6. Why is the Sunshine policy important in inter-Korean sports exchanges?

7. Provide an example of how the North Korean government used sport as a tool for achieving its political goals during the 2014 Incheon Asian Games.

8. Explain how inter-Korean sport exchanges may help expand our perspective on global sport diplomacy.

REFERENCES

Allison, L. (1993). *The changing politics of sport*. Manchester, UK: Manchester University Press.

Armstrong, C. K. (2005). Familism, socialism and political religion in North Korea. *Totalitarian Movements and Political Religions 6*, 383-394.

Bae, J-Y.,& Myong, S. (2011). South Korea's foreign policy toward Korean issues: The feasibility for independent variable and its limits. *Korea and World Politics, 27*(4), 40-42.

BBC. (2000, June 15). North-South joint declaration.[Website]. http://news.bbc.co.uk/2/hi/asia-pacific/791691.stm

Borowiec, Steven. (September 2014). Tensions between North and South Korea at Incheon's Asian Games 2014. *The Guardian*. Retrieved from http://www.theguardian.com/world/2014/sep/18/tensions-north-south-korea-incheon-asian-games

Chang, K. S. (1999). Compressed modernity and its discontents: South Korea society in transition. *Economy and Society, 28*, 30-55.

Chung, D-S. (1998). *Sports and Politics*. Seoul, South Korea: Saram & Saram.

Funabashi, Y. (2007). *The peninsula questions: A chronicle of the second Korean nuclear crisis*. Washington, DC: Brookings Institution Press.

Ha, W-Y. (1998). Korean sports in the 1980s and the Seoul Olympic Games of 1988. *Journal of Olympic History, 6*(2), 11-13.

Harrision, S. S. (2003). *Korean endgame: A strategy for reunification and U.S. disengagement*. Princeton, NJ: Princeton University Press.

Heo, U.,& Roehrig, T. (2014). *South Korea's rise: Economic development, power, and foreign relations*. Cambridge, UK: Cambridge University Press.

Hill, C. R. (1996). *Olympic politics*. Manchester, UK: Manchester University Press.

Hoberman, J. (1984). *Sports and political ideology*. Austin, TX: University of Texas Press.

Houlihan, B. (2007). Politics and sport. In J. Coakley & E. Dunning (Eds.) *Handbook of sports studies* pp. 213-227. London, UK: Sage.

Jackson, S. J. (2013). The contested terrain of sport diplomacy in a globalizing world. *International Area Studies Review, 16*, 274-284.

Jeon, Y. S. (2006). The necessities and direction of developing unification culture contents in Korea. *Korea Cultural Research, 18,* 23-27.

Josson, G. (2006). *Towards Korean reconciliation: Socio-cultural exchanges and cooperation.* Hampshire, UK: Ashgate Publishing Limited.

Jung, G. (2013). Sport as a catalyst for cooperation: Why sport dialogue between the two Koreas succeeds in some cases but not in others. *International Area Studies Review, 16,* 307-324.

Kim, C. I. E. (1962). Japanese rule in Korea (1905-1910). *Proceedings of the American Philosophical Society, 106,* 53-59.

Kim, I. S., Kim, Y. Y., Lee, S. H. & Yu, S. E. (2014). The promotion project on sociocultural exchange and communication between North and South Koreans. *Advanced Science and Technology Letters, 66,* 32-37.

Korean Ministry of Unification (2008, July 4). History of inter-Korean relations: Key points in the South-North Joint Communiqué. February 25, 2008. Retrieved from http://eng.unikorea.go.kr/content.do?cmsid=1806

Korean Ministry of Unification. (2015). Chronology of inter-Korean dialogue. [Website]. Retrieved from http://eng.unikorea.go.kr/content.do?cmsid=3034

Lee, H-R. (2002). Talks and prospects for building sport infrastructure for national unification. *The Journal of Sports and Law, 3,* 165-182.

Lee, J. W. (2010). The Olympics in the post-soviet era: The case of the two Koreas. In A. Bairner & G. Molnar (Eds.) *The politics of the Olympics: A survey,* (117-128). Abingdon: Routledge.

Lee, J. W. (2015). Do the scale and scope of the event matter? The Asian Games and the relations between North and South Korea. *Sport and Society.* Retrieved from http://dx.doi.org/10.1080/17430437.2015.1088723

Lim, J-C. (2012). North Korea's hereditary succession comparing two key transitions in the DPRK. *Asian Survey 52,* 550-570.

Markel, U. (2008). The politics of sport diplomacy and reunification in divided Korea: One nation, two countries and three flags. *International Review for the Sociology of Sport 43,* 289-311.

Markel, U. (2009). Sport, politics and reunification: A comparative analysis of Korea and Germany. *The International Journal of the History of Sport, 26,* 406-428.

Marks, J. (1998). The French national team and national identity: Cette France d'un 'bleu metis'. *Sport in Society, 1*(2), 41-57.

Moon, C-I. (2002), The sunshine policy and the Korean summit: Assessments and prospects. In T. Akaha (Ed) *The future of North Korea* (pp. 26-46). London, UK: Routledge.

Rhee, K-S. (1993). Korea's unification: The applicability of the German experience. *Asian Survey 33,* 360-375.

Snyder, S. (2005). South Korea's squeeze play. *The Washington Quarterly, 28*(4), 93-106.

ABOUT THE EDITORS

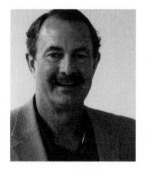

CRAIG ESHERICK is an associate professor at George Mason University. He is the Associate Director of the Center for Sport Management at Mason, where he has engaged in a cooperative agreement with the U.S. Department of State, SportsUnited and the Sport Visitors program for the last five years. Besides this work as a sport diplomat he also participated in the Summer Olympics in 1988 in Seoul, Korea as an assistant coach for the U.S. Men's Olympic basketball team. Before his move to academia, Craig was a basketball player and a basketball coach at Georgetown University, where he earned degrees in finance (BSBA) and law (JD).

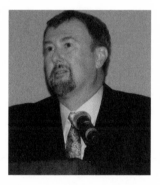

DR. ROBERT BAKER is a professor and director of the Center for Sport Management and Division of Sport Recreation and Tourism at George Mason University. He earned his doctorate from the College of William & Mary, and his M.S. and B.S. from Penn State University. He has served as president of the North American Society for Sport Management, as a founding commissioner of the Commission on Sport Management Accreditation and a founding board member of the World Association of Sport Management. Dr. Baker received NASSM's 2010 Distinguished Sport Management Educator Award and NASPE's 2011 Outstanding Achievement in Sport Management Award. In addition to numerous books and articles, Dr. Baker has served as principal investigator on over $6 million in grants supporting sport diplomacy projects.

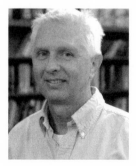

STEVE JACKSON is a professor at the University of Otago, New Zealand. He obtained a BA (Honors) degree from Western University (Ontario, Canada) and his MSc and PhD from the University of Illinois, Urbana-Champaign. In addition to his post at Otago Steve has served as a visiting professor at Charles University (Czech Republic), the University of Jyvaskyla (Finland), the University of British Columbia (Canada), the National Taiwan Normal University and the University of Johannesburg (South Africa). Steve's publications include: *The Other Sport Mega-Event: Rugby World Cup 2011* (Routledge); *The Contested Terrain of the New Zealand All Blacks: Rugby, Commerce, and Cultural Politics in the Age of Globalisation* (Peter Lang); *Sport, Beer, and Gender: Promotional Culture and*

Contemporary Social Life (Peter Lang); and *Sport and Foreign Policy in a Globalising World* (Routledge). Steve is a past-president of the International Sociology of Sport Association (ISSA) and a former New Zealand national ice hockey team player and coach.

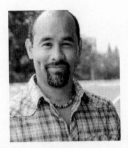 MICHAEL SAM is a senior lecturer in the School of Physical Education, Sport and Exercise Sciences at the University of Otago (New Zealand). His research encompasses policy, politics and governance as they relate to the public administration and management of sport. Dr. Sam has published widely in both sport studies and parent discipline journals and has co-edited two books: *Sport in the City: Cultural Connections* (2011) and *Sport Policy in Small States* (2016). Mike serves on the editorial board of the *International Journal of Sport* Policy and Politics and is the general secretary of the International Sociology of Sport Association (ISSA).

ABOUT THE AUTHORS

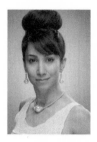

Soolmaz Abooali is a scholar and practitioner who brings the dimension of sport to social change. She is a PhD candidate at George Mason University, studying the ways in which sport is used for conflict resolution. Ms. Abooali is an 11-time U.S. National Karate champion and international medalist, representing the USA around the world. She serves as an athlete ambassador for the American Amateur Karate Federation, and Shirzanan, a media and advocacy platform for Muslim women in sport. Ms. Abooali designs programs related to sport diplomacy and conflict resolution for diverse audiences including government, nonprofit, and philanthropic organizations.

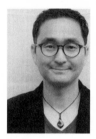

Ik Young Chang is a research associate in the New Zealand Centre for Sport Policy and Politics at the University of Otago and a lecturer at Korea National Sport University (KNSU), South Korea. Prior to obtaining his PhD from the University of Otago, he secured bachelors and master's degrees in physical education at KNSU. He subsequently moved to Canada to complete a second master's degree (Kinesiology) at Lakehead University supported by a South Korean government scholarship. His research primarily focuses on sport and the politics of identity within the contexts of transnational migration and has been published in the *International Review for the Sociology of Sport, International Journal of Sport Communication* and the *Journal of Korean Sociology of Sport*.

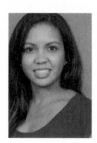

Alicia Cintron is an assistant professor in the School of Human Services at the University of Cincinnati. Her primary research interests surround professional sport facility financing and public policy. Prior to completing her graduate studies at the University of Louisville, Alicia worked in facility management, where she held the positions of assistant marketing manager at UCF Arena in Orlando, Florida, and director of marketing at the Ted Constant Convocation Center in Norfolk, Virginia.

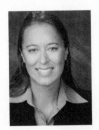

Dr. Jenn Jacobs is a visiting assistant professor in the Department of Kinesiology and Physical Education at Northern Illinois University where she also serves as the assistant director of the Physical Activity and Life Skills (PALS) Group. Dr. Jacobs's scholarship is focused on sport-based youth development, specifically how life skills can be learned through sport experiences. She served as a consultant on the Belizean Youth Sport Coalition (BYSC) project, managing content related to sport psychology and program evaluation.

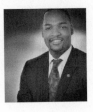

Omari Faulkner a trailblazing cultural and sports diplomacy champion with a ten-year track record of remarkable success within the field. Mr. Faulkner's exemplary global service has earned him national recognition and two prestigious distinctions, the State Department Recognition Award, presented by former Secretary of State Colin Powell and the State Department Superior Honor Award. Mr. Faulkner is the founder and president of O Street International, a nonprofit organization focused primarily on sports and cultural diplomacy. He also serves as an adjunct professor within Georgetown University's Sport Industry Management program.

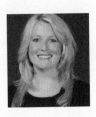

Melissa Ferry is a sport leadership doctoral student in the Center for Sport Leadership at Virginia Commonwealth University. She completed her MEd in Sport Leadership at VCU, and received her BSEd in physical education at George Mason University, where she was a co-captain of the women's track and field team. Her research focuses on gender equity issues in athletics, specifically the lack of women in coaching, as well as athletic administration. She serves on the Virginia High School League Coaching Education committee, and was a head coach of girls track and field at Fairfax County Public Schools. Prior to working on her doctorate, she previously taught secondary health and physical education for seven years with Fairfax County Public Schools.

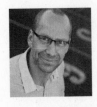

Jonathan Grix is a reader in sport policy and politics in the School of Sport, Exercise and Rehabilitation Sciences and director of the Sport Policy Centre at the University of Birmingham. He has published widely in the area of sport and politics. His latest monographs include *Sport under Communism: Behind the East German "Miracle"* (co-authored with Mike Dennis) (Palgrave, 2012) and *Sport Politics: An Introduction* (Palgrave, 2016). Jonathan is the editor-in-chief of the *International Journal of Sport Policy and Politics* published by Taylor and Francis.

Bob Heere is an associate professor and PhD program director in the Department of Sport and Entertainment at the University of South Carolina. Prior to joining SPTE, he held academic appointments at the University of Texas at Austin, Florida State University, The Cruyff Institute for Sport Studies, and Auckland University of Technology. His research expertise is on the social impact of sport on society, with a particular focus on social identity theory and community development. To that end, he has conducted research on five different continents, cooperating with researchers from China, Korea, Japan, New Zealand, Aruba, Serbia, United Kingdom, Spain, Germany, Belgium, Netherlands, Brazil and South Africa. His research has been published in leading sport management journals such as *Journal of Sport Management, Sport Management Review, European Sport Management Quarterly* and *Sport Marketing Quarterly.*

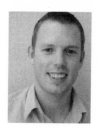

Dr. Steven M. Howell is an assistant professor in the Department of Kinesiology and Physical Education at Northern Illinois University where he also serves as an associate director of the Physical Activity and Life Skills (PALS) Group. Broadly speaking, Howell's research centers on examining the extent to which policy and policy changes inform and impact practice within the context of sport. More specifically, one of his interests is on investigating and evaluating outreach initiatives utilizing sport for social change and development. As described in this book, Howell served as a policy consultant and statistician on the Belizean Youth Sport Coalition (BYSC) project.

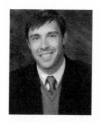

Scott R. Jedlicka is an assistant professor of sport management at Washington State University. His research focuses on sport governance and developing theoretical explanations of its relationship to public and foreign policy. Scott's work has been published in the *International Journal of the History of Sport* and the *International Journal of Sport Policy and Politics.* He and his wife Cara reside in Pullman, Washington.

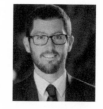

Tim Kellison is an assistant professor in the Department of Kinesiology and Health at Georgia State University. His primary research interests are organizational theory and public policy. Within these fields, his research has focused on the politics of sport facility financing, urban and regional planning, and environmentally sustainable design. The unifying theme of his scholarship is the study of the ways in which sport organizations act as community leaders with respect to various sociopolitical issues. His work has been published in peer-reviewed journals including the

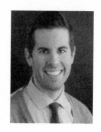

Journal of Sport Management, Sport Management Review, and *European Sport Management Quarterly.* Additionally, his research has been referenced in *The New York Times, National Public Radio, ESPN The Magazine, Atlanta Journal-Constitution,* and *Tampa Bay Times.*

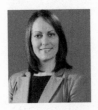

Carrie LeCrom, Ph.D., is the executive director of the Center for Sport Leadership at Virginia Commonwealth University, where she has taught since 2005. She is passionate about the use of sport for social change, and has generated over $650,000 in grant funding from sources such as the U.S. Department of State and the NCAA. Much of her work is focused on increasing cultural understanding and combatting other social issues abroad through the intentional use of sport. Her research interests focus on sport for development, global sport, and sport consumer behavior. She was the recipient of the 2014 Ruch Award for Excellence in Teaching and the 2016 Award of Excellence, both given by the VCU School of Education.

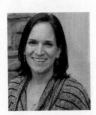

Dr. Laura Misener is associate professor in the School of Kinesiology at Western University in London, Ontario. Her research focuses on how sport and events can be used as instruments of social change. Her work critically examines numerous ways that sport events have been purported to positively influence community development, social infrastructure, social inclusion, and healthy lifestyles of community members. Dr. Misener's current research program is focusing on the role of sport events for persons with a disability in influencing community accessibility and perceptions of disability. Her work on events and urban community development has been published in scholarly outlets such as *Journal of Sport Management, Journal of Organization and Management, Managing Leisure,* and *Journal of Sport and Social Issues.* She co-edited a special issue of Sport Management Review on Managing Disability Sport, and is currently an Associate Editor of Leisure Sciences.

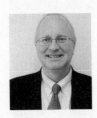

Dr. Robert Orttung is research director at the George Washington University Sustainability Collaborative and associate research professor of International Affairs at GW's Elliott School of International Affairs. He is the author or editor of numerous books and articles about Russian politics. With Sufian Zhemukhov, he is the co-author of the forthcoming book, *The 2014 Winter Olympics and the Evolution of Putin's Russia.*

Dr. Jim Ressler is an associate professor in the Department of Kinesiology and Physical Education at Northern Illinois University. Dr. Ressler's scholarship is focused on pedagogical approaches to teaching and learning in physical education, and school-university partnerships in teacher preparation. His primary interests include adventure-based learning (ABL) as a pedagogical approach and the import of personal and social development for all learners. He was the co-principal investigator and facilitator on the Belizean Youth Sport Coalition (BYSC) project, managing content related to effective planning and instructional strategies.

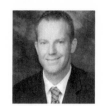

Kyle Rich is a PhD candidate at Western University in London, Ontario, Canada. He is interested in the social aspects of sport and recreation management, particularly in relation to community development. Kyle's research has examined sport and recreation in a variety of contexts, including rural communities, national water safety programs, and local sport for social inclusion initiatives. He is also interested in participatory approaches to research and how research activities can be useful in and for communities.

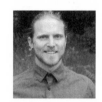

Dr. Claudio M. Rocha is an assistant professor at the School of Physical Education and Sport of Ribeirao Preto – University of Sao Paulo. He received his doctorate from the Ohio State University, with a major in sport management and a minor in research methods. During his doctoral studies, he was fully funded by the Fulbright Commission and Brazilian Ministry of Education. In the 2014-2015 academic year, Dr. Rocha was a visiting scholar at Isenberg School of Management, University of Massachusetts – Amherst. His research has been published in top sport management journals, such as *Journal of Sport Management* and *European Sport Management Quarterly,* and in top leisure journals, such as *Leisure Studies.* Dr. Rocha has recently contributed to three chapters in two books: *Sport in Latin America* (2016) and *Routledge Handbook of Sport Management* (2012). His current research interests are in legacies of sport mega-events hosted by developing nations and international sport consumption behavior.

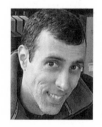

Myles J. Schrag has a master's of science degree in kinesiology with a sociocultural emphasis from University of Illinois at Urbana-Champaign, where his thesis was on sport and peace-building. He has been an editor of sport and exercise science books for 16 years, is the author of two books on sport history, and is a freelance writer. He writes a blog on sport, spirituality, and service issues.

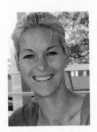

Judit Trunkos is a PhD student at the University of South Carolina with the first field of international relations and second field of comparative politics. In terms of research interests, Judit has been examining soft power, more specifically culture's influence on foreign policy choices. In comparative politics, her focus has been the democratization and political culture of European countries. Prior to attending USC, Judit has completed her master's at Winthrop University focusing on the new tools of diplomacy in the 21st century. Her publications include topics such as the conceptual development of soft power and Russia's reliance on soft and hard power instruments.

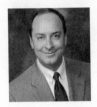

Dr. Paul M. Wright is the Lane/Zimmerman Endowed professor in the Department of Kinesiology and Physical Education at Northern Illinois University where he also serves as the director of the Physical Activity and Life Skills (PALS) Group. Dr. Wright's scholarship is focused on positive youth development through sport and physical activity. He is a Fulbright Scholar and internationally recognized expert on the Teaching Personal and Social Responsibility (TPSR) instructional model. He was the principal investigator on the Belizean Youth Sport Coalition (BYSC) project, described in this book, which was funded by the SportsUnited program of the U.S. Department of State to promote youth development and social change through sport in Belize.

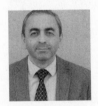

Sufian Zhemukhov (PhD, Russian Academy of Science's Institute of Ethnology and Anthropology, 1997) is senior research associate at The George Washington University's Institute for European, Russian and Eurasian Studies and Adjunct Professor at the University of Maryland, Baltimore County. He was a Kennan-Fulbright Scholar (2005-2006), a Heyward Isham Fellow at The George Washington University (2011-2012), and a Charles H. Revson Foundation Fellow at the US Holocaust Memorial Museum and Scholar Rescue Fund (2012). His research interests include nationalism, Islam, ethnic relations and politics. His academic articles appeared in *Slavic Review, East European Politics, Problems of Post-Communism, Nationalities Papers, and Religion, State & Society,* among others.

INDEX